新起航大学英语系列教材

根据最新《大学英语教学指南》编写

医护英语
Medical English

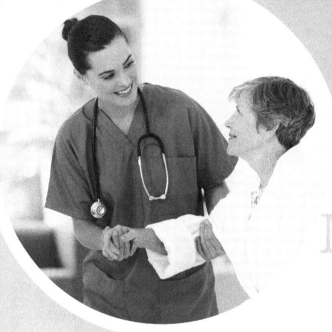

主　编　周桂香

副主编　梁丽燕　覃德英

编　者　唐季红　李贺静　陈宜凝

　　　　艾为珍　姜怡佳　黄　智

　　　　何　芸

MEDICAL

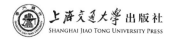

上海交通大学出版社

SHANGHAI JIAO TONG UNIVERSITY PRESS

内容提要

本书编写的根本出发点是培养适合社会及岗位需求的应用型护理技术人才。本书结合护理专业学生毕业后的工作实际,力求为他们提供未来工作岗位所需的英语知识,从而达到护理专业学生涉外英语交流无障碍的目的。本书主体部分的英文课文主要介绍护理理论知识并辅以对话,配有临床护理工作中基础护理操作的应用及常见护理操作技能,兼顾英语语言学习和职业操作技能培养,将大学英语教学与医护专业知识紧密结合,全面提高学习者在护理实际工作中的英语综合运用能力。

本书共有 9 个单元,涵盖了医学院校护理学主要教授的理论及临床知识,单元主题按照护理程序、病人入院、检查生命体征、给药、内科、外科、妇科、儿科、病人出院的顺序来编排。最后本书还附有全国医护英语等级考试(METS)的样卷,为有志参加该考试的学习者提供参考。

图书在版编目(CIP)数据

医护英语/周桂香主编.—上海:上海交通大学出版社,2020
ISBN 978-7-313-21544-4

Ⅰ.①医… Ⅱ.①周… Ⅲ.①医学—英语—医学院校—教材
Ⅳ.①R

中国版本图书馆 CIP 数据核字(2019)第 134382 号

医护英语
YIHU YINGYU

主　　编:	周桂香		
出版发行:	上海交通大学出版社	地　　址:	上海市番禺路 951 号
邮政编码:	200030	电　　话:	021-64071208
印　　制:	苏州市古得堡数码印刷有限公司	经　　销:	全国新华书店
开　　本:	787mm×1092mm　1/16	印　　张:	9
字　　数:	222 千字		
版　　次:	2020 年 7 月第 1 版	印　　次:	2020 年 7 月第 1 次印刷
书　　号:	ISBN 978-7-313-21544-4	ISBN 978-7-88941-276-6	
定　　价:	39.00 元		

前　言

　　本书编写的根本出发点是培养适合社会及岗位需求的应用型护理技术人才。本书结合护理专业学生毕业后的工作实际,力求为他们提供未来工作岗位所需的英语知识,从而达到护理专业学生涉外英语交流无障碍的目的。本书主体部分的英文课文主要介绍护理理论知识并辅以对话,配有临床护理工作中基础护理操作的应用及常见护理操作技能,兼顾英语语言学习和职业操作技能培养,将大学英语教学与医护专业知识紧密结合,全面提高学习者在护理实际工作中的英语综合运用能力。

　　本书共有 9 个单元,涵盖了医学院校护理学主要教授的理论及临床知识,单元主题按照护理程序、病人入院、检查生命体征、给药、内科、外科、妇科、儿科、病人出院的顺序来编排。每个单元有三个部分:一篇主课文、一个情景对话以及与单元主题相关的护理操作技术,如铺床、生命体征、注射、插胃管、导尿、无菌操作、吸氧等。主课文的知识难度适中,附有参考译文及生词表;情景对话部分围绕特定的专题展开,有利于学生模仿并学以致用;护理操作流程清晰易懂,并辅以实用的护理用语,扩充了临床护理实践技能。最后本书还附有全国医护英语等级考试(METS)的样卷,为有志参加该考试的学习者提供参考。

　　本教材编写组成员认真搜集素材,经仔细审阅并不断修改完善后才最终定稿。在此过程中,得到了护理专业教师的指导以及院校同行的帮助,在此表示由衷感谢! 由于时间仓促及编写者护理专业知识有限,本教材存在的不足之处,真诚欢迎广大师生和读者批评指正。

编者

2020 年 3 月

CONTENTS

CONTENTS

Unit 1

Nursing Process

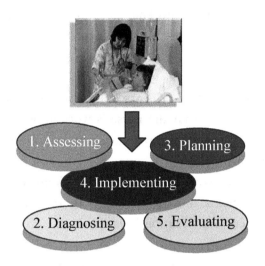

Part Ⅰ Text

Warming-up

1. What is the nursing process?
2. What are the steps of the nursing process?
3. What is the use of the nursing process in nursing?

Topic-related Terms

Match the words in Column A with their meanings in Column B.

Column A	Column B
1. assessment	a. diagnose（What is the problem?）
2. diagnosis	b. assess（What data is collected?）
3. planning	c. plan（How to manage the problem?）
4. implementation	d. evaluate（Does the plan work?）
5. evaluation	e. putting plan into action

1

Nursing Process

What is the nursing process? In nursing, this process is one of the foundations of practice. It offers a framework for thinking through problems and provides some organization to a nurse's critical thinking skills. It's important to point out that this process is flexible and not rigid. It is a tool to use in nursing care.

The nursing process is a scientific method used by nurses to ensure the quality of patient care. This approach can be broken down into five separate steps. Here is an acronym to help you: **ADPIE**, which stands for assessing, diagnosing, planning, implementing and evaluating.①

Assessing

The first step in the nursing process is assessing. In this phase, data is gathered about the patient, family or community that the nurse is working with. Objective data, or data that can be collected through examination, is measurable.② This includes things like vital signs or observable patient behaviors.

Subjective data is gathered from patients as they talk about their needs, feelings, and perspectives about the problems they're having.③ In this step, information about the patient's response to their current situation is established.

Diagnosing

The second phase of the nursing process is diagnosing. The nurse takes the information from the assessment, analyzes the information, and identifies problems where patient outcomes can be improved through the use of nursing interventions.④

Planning

The third phase of the nursing process is planning. The nurse prioritizes which diagnoses need to be focused on. The patient can, and should, be involved in this process. Planning starts with identifying patient goals. Goals are statements of what needs to be accomplished and stem from the diagnoses—both short and long term goals should be established. Next, the nurse plans the steps needed to reach those goals, and an individualized plan with related nursing interventions is created.

Implementing

The fourth phase of the nursing process, implementing, occurs when the nursing interventions, or plan, are actually carried out.

Common nursing interventions include pain management, preventing complications following surgery, teaching and educating patients, and procedures that are part of nursing care.

Evaluating

Once all nursing intervention actions have taken place, the nurse completes an evaluation to determine of the goals for patient wellness to be met. The possible patient outcomes are generally described under three terms: patient's condition improved, patient's condition stabilized，and patient's condition deteriorated，died，or discharged. ⑤ In the event the condition of the patient has shown no improvement，or if the wellness goals are not met，the nursing process begins again from the first step.

All nurses must be familiar with the steps of the nursing process. If you're planning on studying to become a nurse，be prepared to use these phases everyday in your new career.

Words and Expressions

acronym/ˈækrənɪm/ n . 首字母缩略词

deteriorate/dɪˈtɪərɪəreɪt/ v . 使恶化

discharge/dɪsˈtʃɑːdʒ/ vt . 下(客)；卸船；免除(自己的义务、负担等)；执行

　　　　　 vt .& vi . 放出；流出；开枪；发射

　　　　　 n .(气体、液体如水从管子里)流出；排放出的物体

implement/ˈɪmplɪmənt/ v . 实施,执行；使生效,实现；落实(政策)；把……填满

objective/əbˈdʒektɪv/ adj . 目标的；客观的

perspective/pəˈspektɪv/ n . 观点,看法,远景,景色；洞察力

prioritize/praɪˈɒrətaɪz/ v . 优先处理；按重要性排列,划分优先顺序

subjective/səbˈdʒektɪv/ adj . 主观的；个人的

break...down into 分成不同种类；分解成……

stem from 出于；来自,起源于,由……造成

Notes

① 缩写 ADPIE 可以帮助你记住护理程序的五个步骤,ADPIE 五个字母分别代表评估、诊断、计划、实施和评价。

② 客观数据或通过体检收集来的数据是可以测量的。

③ 主观数据是通过交流收集到病人生病时的需求、感受和想法。

④ 护士通过护理评估收集信息、分析信息、找出问题,并运用护理干预改善患者病情。这里 where 引导的是定语从句。

⑤ 病人的结果一般可以描述成这三种情况：病情好转了；病情稳定了；因病情恶化,病人死亡或出院了。

Text Exploration

Decide whether the following sentence is true or false. If it is true，put "T" in the bracket，if it is false，put "F" in the bracket.

1. Multiple diagnoses are sometimes made for a single patient. (　　)

2. The third phase of the nursing process doesn't start with identifying patient goals. (　　)

3. Implementation of the nursing process occurs when the nursing interventions，or plan，are actually carried out. (　　)

4. An evaluation is completed to determine of the goals for patient wellness to be met as

soon as all nursing intervention actions have taken place. (   )

5. Patients' feelings and perspectives about the problems they're having are objective data. (   )

Part Ⅱ Dialogue

Read the following dialogue. Then do the Role-play task by using the Sentence Models with your partner.

(A nurse is getting information from a patient)

Nurse：Good afternoon! Your name is Li Hua, right?

Li Hua：Yes, what's the matter?

Nurse：Would you mind my asking you some questions?

Li Hua：Please go ahead.

Nurse：What's your height?

Li Hua：I am 159 centimeters tall.

Nurse：What about your weight?

Li Hua：69 kilograms.

Nurse：What's the problem?

Li Hua：I have a pain in my abdomen.

Nurse：How long have you had it?

Li Hua：It started in the morning. At the beginning I had a stomachache.

Nurse：How long did it last?

Li Hua：About three hours. But this afternoon it moved to the right lower part of the abdomen.

Nurse：Have you had any other symptoms?

Li Hua：I have had nausea.

Nurse：Have you had any diarrhea?

Li Hua：No.

Nurse：Any fever?

Li Hua：I don't know.

Nurse：Let me take your temperature. All right，you have a slight fever. Please lie down on the bed. I'll ask the doctor to examine your abdomen. Don't be nervous and try to relax.

Li Hua：All right.

Words and Expressions

abdomen/ˈæbdəmən/ *n*. 腹部；腹腔；下腹；［虫］腹部

stomachache/ˈstʌməkeɪk/ *n*. 胃痛；腹痛

symptom/ˈsɪmptəm/ *n*. 症状；征兆

nausea/ˈnɔːzɪə/ *n*. 恶心;反胃;作呕;极度厌恶

diarrhea/ˌdaɪəˈrɪə/ *n*. 腹泻

Sentence Models

Would you mind my asking you some questions?

What's your height?

How long have you had it?

Have you had any other symptoms?

Have you had any diarrhea?

Role-play

Make an communication with a patient. Student A acts as a patient; student B acts as a nurse who is going to communicate with the patient.

Use the above Sentence Models as guidelines.

Part Ⅲ　Scene Practice

Read the information about nursing process. The nursing process can be a confusing concept for nursing students to grasp. Below is an example of the process from start to finish in a story like fashion.

Assessment

John visits his general physician on Monday because he was feeling sick over the weekend. When he is called back from the waiting room, the nurse on staff takes his temperature, heart rate, and blood pressure. She then asks John a series of questions about how he's been feeling lately. The nurse notes his responses when he says he's been having difficulty breathing and has been feeling very tired. She also sees on John's medical history that he has had previous problems with his cholesterol levels and blood pressure. John also has a blood sample taken during his doctor's visit.

Diagnosis

The nurse looks over John's symptoms and notes that his heart-rate is higher than average and his blood pressure is elevated. She also considers that he's experienced fatigue and shortness of breath before when his cholesterol levels were very high. The nurse determines that John is experiencing hyperlipidemia, also known as having high levels of fat within the blood. John's blood tests confirm this hypothesis. The nurse is also concerned that John is at risk for heart disease.

Planning

John returns on Tuesday for a follow-up visit. The nurse sits down with him in a closed room and explains his cholesterol levels and high blood pressure. She suggests that John be put on medication to help lower these numbers and recommends he exercise at least twice a week. The nurse also tells John he should stay away from salty foods and eat less red meat. John agrees with the nurse, and they setup a follow-up appointment two weeks later. The nurse reminds John to call if there are any changes in his condition, or if he starts to feel worse.

Implementation

John is prescribed the medication and takes it as recommended. One week later, he has a day when he feels especially sick and calls the doctor's office. The nurse explains that the medication could cause nausea as a side-effect and advises John to drink ginger ale and avoid any foods that generally upset his stomach. John continues taking the medication and goes to the gym four times during the two week period. Once the two weeks has passed, he returns to the doctor's office for his follow-up appointment.

Evaluation

When John returns, the nurse asks him a series of questions about how he's been feeling. John replies that he has been having an easier time breathing and feels significantly less tired since exercising and taking the medication. The nurse marks "Patient's Condition Improved" on his official medical records and congratulates John on his well being. She then advises him to remain on the medication for one more month and to continue his exercise.

Although there are calculated steps behind the nurse's approach, her methods are extremely friendly and warming and care is taken to treat the patient like a human being. As you can see, the nursing process will feel like second nature when put into real-world practice.

Words and Expressions

hyperlipidemia/ˈhaɪpəlɪpɪˈdiːmɪə/ n. 血脂过多,高脂血症;高血脂

cholesterol/kəˈlestərɒl/ n. 胆固醇

elevate/ˈelɪveɪt/ v. 提高;提升

hypothesis/haɪˈpɒθəsɪs/ n. 假设;前提

a follow-up visit 随访

nausea/ˈnɔːzɪə/ v. 恶心;反胃;作呕;极度厌恶

ginger ale/ˌdʒɪndʒə ˈeɪl/ n. 姜汁无酒精饮料;姜汁汽水;干姜水;姜汁啤酒

calculated/ˈkælkjʊleɪtɪd/ adj. 计算出的;有计划的;适当的;适合

Critical Thinking

Work in pairs and discuss the following questions.

1. To clarify the nursing diagnosis, what should a nurse do?
2. What recommendations should a nurse give a patient like John for his recovery?
3. What's the nursing process according to your understanding?
4. What's the difference between medical diagnosis and nursing diagnosis?

Unit 2

Admission

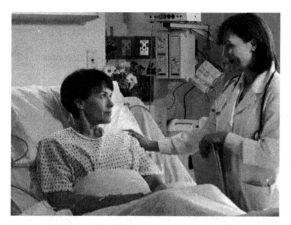 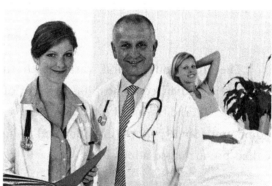

Part I Text

Warming-up

1. What are the main ways in which patients are admitted to hospital?
2. How can patients effectively prevent cross-infection?
3. To ensure a peaceful and healthy recovery environment, what should the patients do?

Topic-related Terms

Match the words in Column A with their meanings in Column B.

Column A	Column B
1. admission	a. separate part or room in a hospital for a particular group of patients
2. schedule	b. work together
3. infection	c. an unexpected and difficult situation, especially an accident, which happens suddenly and which requires quick action to deal with it

（续表）

4. attendant	d. plan, organize, and carry out (an event)
5. emergency	e. an ordered list of times at which things are planned to occur
6. arrangement	f. entering or being allowed to enter a building, hospital, etc.
7. ward	g. the invasion of the body by pathogenic microorganisms and their multiplication which can lead to tissue damage and disease
8. cooperate	h. someone who waits on or tends to or attends to the needs of another

Admission①

The admission method varies with the different condition of the patients. Some patients are admitted to hospital because of accidents or sudden illnesses. They are often seriously ill and in need of immediate care and attention. This is called emergency admission. Some patients are admitted to hospital for diseases, which are not acute. This is called pre-arranged admission.

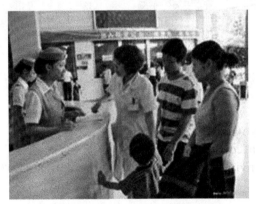 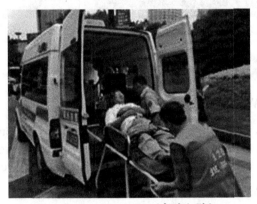

pre-arranged admissions（常规入院）   emergency admissions（急症入院）

Whether you are admitted to hospital for pre-arranged or emergency admission, to guarantee your pleasant stay during your hospitalization, I would like to take a few moments to make a brief introduction on the safety notes you might need to know during your hospitalization. ②

1. Ward Environment

Each patient room is equipped with patient's bed, beeper, bathroom, television, air-conditioner, cabinet, bed stand, and thermos.

2. Patient's Schedule

Please kindly follow our treatment schedule as provided below：

Time	Agenda
7: 00 a.m.	Keep an empty stomach if our nurse needs to take your blood sample. Please collect your own urine and stool sample in the container provided before 7: 00 a.m. ③
8: 30 a.m.	The ward rounds and treatment start at 8: 30 a.m. Please remain in the room at the same time. (Please finish your breakfast before 8: 30 a.m.)
12: 00 p.m.	Lunch time
15: 00 p.m. – 19: 30 p.m.	Visiting hours
18: 00 p.m.	Dinner time
21: 30 p.m. – 22: 00 p.m.	Bed time (Please turn off your room's light or television to keep a quite environment in our hospital)

3. Help Us to Prevent Infection

Let us work together to maintain a healthy environment and to avoid infection.

We have clean-keeping attendants to maintain a clean environment every day. However, we can make this a better environment if you work together with us.

a) Wash your hands regularly. Make sure you use a soap in a right way when washing your hands.

b) Do not smoke. Smoking is strictly prohibited in our hospital. Not only will it affect your health but also the people around you.

c) Cover your mouth and nose when you cough or sneeze to avoid germ-spreading.

d) Inform our medical staff if you have ever caught a flu or fever.

e) Avoid spitting to keep our environment clean.

4. Patient Responsibilities

To ensure a peaceful and healthy recovery environment, we would simply ask you to cooperate with us.

a) Please try to keep your voice down in the ward and keep a minimum volume when using your television or computer.

b) Do not smoke or drink alcohol during your stay.

c) Please conserve water and electricity.

d) Please keep clean of our wards' environment.

e) Please take care of your belongings during your stay.

f) Please make proper use of the equipment we provide and avoid vandalism as any damaged equipment will be charged accordingly. ④

5. Meal

We serve a variety of Chinese, Muslim, and Western food. When you need special diets, our clinical dietitian is available. If you don't want to eat in the hospital and need to order food from outside，please contact our customer service for assistance.

6. Outing

If you need to travel outside the hospital，please kindly seek for your doctor for travelling permission.

7. Patient Rights

Patients have the right to express any concern about their treatment. We will thank you for addressing your concerns immediately to our customer service so that we can respond as quickly as possible. ⑤

Words and Expression

admission/æd'mɪʃən/ n . 入院，准许进入

procedure/prə'siːdʒə(r)/ n . 程序，手续

emergency/ɪ'mɜːdʒənsɪ/ n . 紧急情况；突发事件；非常时刻
                     adj . 紧急的，应急的

guarantee/ˌgærən'tiː/ n . 保证，担保；保证人，保证书；抵押品
                 v . 保证，担保

hospitalization/ˌhɒspɪtəlaɪ'zeɪʃən/ n . 医院收容，住院治疗；送入医院；留诊

ward/wɔːd/ n . 病房，病室

agenda/ə'dʒendə/ n . 日常工作事项；议程

infection/ɪn'fekʃən/ n . 〈医〉传染，感染；传染病，染毒物；影响

regularly/'regjələlɪ/ adv . 有规律地，按时，照例，按部就班地

prohibit/prə(ʊ)'hɪbɪt/ vt . 禁止，阻止，防止；不准许

staff/stɑːf/ n . 全体职员

responsibility/rɪˌspɒnsə'bɪlətɪ/ n . 责任；职责；责任感

minimum/'mɪnɪməm/ adj . 最低的；最小的；最少的

vandalism/'vænd(ə)lɪz(ə)m/ n . 故意破坏，捣毁

convenience/kən'viːnɪəns/ n . 方便，便利；便利设施；个人的舒适或利益

Notes

① 病人的病情不同，入院方式也不同。主要有两种：急症入院和常规入院。

② 为了能让您愉快地度过住院这段时间，我想占用您几分钟，给您简单介绍一些您在住院期间需要了解的相关内容。

③ 7:00 之前用已提供的容器收集自己的尿液、粪便样本。

④ 请正确使用医院提供的各种设备，不得故意损坏，如有损坏请照价赔偿。

⑤ 病人有权对我们的工作提出意见或建议，请您及时把意见或建议反馈给我们的病人服务中心，便于我们能尽快采纳或改进。so that 在此引导目的状语从句。

Text Exploration

Decide whether the following sentence is true or false. If it is true，put "T" in the bracket, if it is false, put "F" in the bracket.

1. The ward rounds and treatment start at 8:30 a.m. (   )
2. The hospital serves a variety of Chinese, Buddhism, and Western food. (   )
3. There is no bathroom in the patient room. (   )
4. If the patient damages the equipment in the hospital, he or she will be charged accordingly. (   )
5. Patients have no right to express any concern about their treatment. (   )

Part Ⅱ Dialogue

Read the following dialogue. Then do the Role-play task by using the Sentence Models with your partner.

Nurse: How do you do, Mrs. Green. Welcome to our hospital. I'm the nurse in charge of you during your stay in hospital and you can call me Mary. Hope you will feel at home here.

Patient: Sorry to bother you.

Nurse: Don't mention it. This is my job. I'll bring you to your ward, please follow me. This way, please! This is your bed.

Patient: Will you show me how to use the button on the panel?

Nurse: Of course. The panel on the head of the bed is equipped with a nurse-call system. If you need anything, just press this button, we will come here as soon as possible.

Patient: OK. Is it all right for my husband to stay here with me?

Nurse: Yes, but he has to pay for his bed. We don't think it is necessary. Your condition isn't so serious.

Patient: What about the treatment schedule?

Nurse: Patients usually get up at 6:30 a.m. Breakfast is from 7 o'clock to 8 o'clock. The ward rounds and treatment start at 8:30 a.m. Lunch is at noon. After that you have a nap. Visiting hour is from 3:00 p.m. to 7:30 p.m. Supper is at 6:00 p.m. Bed time is from 9:30 p.m. to 10:00 p.m.

Patient: Good. Sounds reasonable.

Nurse: In order to take better care of you, I need to get some information about your health history for our nursing records. Would you mind if I ask you some questions?

Patient: Of course not.

Nurse: Thank you. First I need to take your vital signs, that's to say, temperature, respirations, heart rate, and pressure. Please put the thermometer under your armpit. OK, thank you. They are normal except for a low-grade fever. What's wrong with you, Mrs. Green?

Patient: I think I've come down with flu.

Nurse: What's your symptom?

Patient: I feel chilly. And I have a terrible headache and a sore throat.

Nurse: Did you go to see a doctor before?

Patient: Yes. He gave me some medicine but I'm afraid they didn't have an effect.

Nurse: Did you have any other disease before, such as heart disease, diabetes, high blood pressure, pneumonitis, asthma, nephritis, psychiatric disease or anything like that?

Patient: No.

Nurse: Have you ever received a surgery?

Patient: No.

Nurse: Are you allergic to any medicine or food?

Patient: No.

Nurse: I need to ask you a few questions about your family history. Are your parents still alive?

Patient: No, they aren't.

Nurse: Sorry, do you know what caused their death?

Patient: My mother died in a car accident and my father died of high blood pressure.

Nurse: Do you feel anything else uncomfortable?

Patient: I also have a stuffy nose.

Nurse: Well, I will inform your doctor now. Here is a bottle of water, and you must drink plenty of water now, at least 2 000 ml a day. And also you should eat a light diet. Keep the skin and your clothes dry all the time.

Patient: No problem!

Nurse: By the way, don't take anything until the blood is drawn tomorrow morning. We'll take some blood from your arm to do some laboratory examinations which can provide more useful information for the treatment of your disease.

Patient: OK.

Nurse: Do some light work, have a happy outlook, wish you to recover soon! If you need any help, please call us. See you later.

Patient: See you.

Words and Expressions

nformation/ˌɪnfəˈmeɪʃən/ n. 信息,数据

temperature/ˈtemprətʃə(r)/ n. 温度;体温;气温

respirations/respəˈreɪʃnz/ n. 〈医〉呼吸(作用),呼吸音

thermometer/θəˈmɒmɪtə(r)/ n. 温度计;体温表

armpit/ˈɑːmpɪt/ n. 腋窝;胳肢窝

feverish/ˈfiːvərɪʃ/ adj. 发烧的,有热病症状的

diabetes/'daɪə'biːtiːz/ *n*.〈医〉糖尿病

pneumonitis/njuːməʊ'naɪtɪs/ *n*.肺炎

asthma/'æsmə/ *n*.〈医〉气喘,哮喘

nephritis/ne'fraɪtɪs/ *n*.肾炎

psychiatric/'saɪkɪ'ætrɪk/ *adj*.精神病学的;精神病治疗的

allergic/ə'lɜːdʒɪk/ *adj*.过敏的;过敏症的

stuffy/'stʌfɪ/ *adj*.闷热的,不通气的

ward rounds 查房

visiting hours 探视时间

heart disease 心脏病

high blood pressure 高血压

Sentence Models

I'm the nurse in charge of you during your stay in hospital.

Hope you will feel at home here.

I need to get some information about your health history for our nursing records.

Would you mind if I ask you some questions?

What's wrong with you?

I think I've come down with flu.

Are you running a temperature?

Are you allergic to any medicine or food?

Wish you to recover soon.

Role-play

Make a dialogue. Student A acts as a patient; student B acts as a nurse who is going to gather student A's information.

Use Sentence Models as guidelines.

Part Ⅲ Scene Practice ....

Read the information below about admission procedures. Make sure about the correct admission procedures. Student A acts as a patient; Student B acts as a nurse and then practice this action. Use the above sentence Models to communicate with each other effectively.

Admission Procedures

1. The patient takes the hospitalization certificate to the ward and the nurse stands up, smiles, warmly welcomes the patient, lets the patient sit down, and provides the patient with a cup of hot water.

2. The responsible nurse prepares the bed within 5 minutes, sends the patient to the ward, and introduces the hospital (doctors and nurses, ward environment, ordering and opening water time, safety systems, valuables storage, pager application, etc.).

3. The responsible nurse fills in the inpatient medical record, hospitalization list card, and bedside card.

4. Complete a physical examination (body temperature, pulse, respiration, blood pressure, weight, etc.).

5. Tell the doctor to view the patient. Treat the patient immediately according to the doctor's advice.

6. The responsible nurse completes the first nursing record within 4 hours, and communicates with the patient within 8 hours to understand the personality, physiological state, and needs of the patient, and implement targeted nursing.

7. The head nurse greets and introduces herself to the patients who are admitted to the hospital during the day within 8 hours, and to the patients who are admitted to the hospital in the evening within 14 hours.

8. Patients who are admitted to the ward for emergency treatment do not need to go through the hospitalization procedures. They are directly escorted into the ward by the green channel with the emergency department medical staff. The admission procedure is to be re-submitted by the family or staff to the hospital.

9. Strictly implement the "eight services" for patients admitted to hospital:

A warm greeting;

A kind address;

A sincere smile;

A neat bed;

A cup of warm boiled water;

A thoughtful introduction of admission to the hospital;

An accurate and standardized admission assessment;

A detailed and comprehensive health mission.

Words and Expressions

certificate/sə'tɪfɪkeɪt(for v.);sə'tɪfɪkɪt(for n.)/vt. 发给证明书；以证书形式授权给……；用证书批准

n. 证书；执照，文凭

environment/ɪn'vaɪrənmənt/n. 环境，外界

examination/ɪɡˌzæmə'neʃən/n. 考试；检查；查问

physiological/fɪzɪə'lɑdʒɪkl/adj. 生理学的，生理的

implement/'ɪmplɪment/vt. 实施，执行；实现，使生效

n. 工具，器具；手段

escort/'eskɔːrt/n. 陪同；护航舰；护卫队；护送者

vt. 护送;陪同;为……护航

submit/səbˈmɪt/*vt.* 使服从;主张;呈递

vi. 提交;服从

Critical Thinking

Work in pairs and discuss the following questions.

1. Briefly describe the admission procedures.

2. Why should the nurse communicate with the patient in time after the patient is admitted to the hospital?

3. What medical examinations do patients take before admission? Why?

4. As a nurse，how do you plan to serve your patients?

Unit 3

Vital Signs

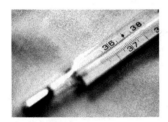 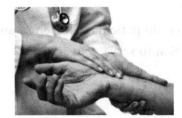 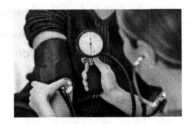

Warming-up

1. What do vital signs include?
2. Why are vital signs measured?
3. What factors will affect vital signs?

Topic-related Terms

Match the words in Column A with their meanings in Column B.

Column A	Column B
1. thermometer	a. difficulty in breathing or shortage of breath
2. axilla	b. one of the tubes that carrying blood from the heart to all parts of the body
3. inhale	c. you use it to measure the patient's temperature
4. inflammation	d. high blood pressure
5. pulse	e. the act of taking air, smoke, etc. into lungs breathing
6. artery	f. the hollow under the shoulder, between the upper arm and the body
7. dyspnea	g. it relates to the normal rhythmical contraction of the heart, during which the blood in the chambers is forced onward

（续表）

8. hypertension	h. it occurs when our body responds to outside stimulation that is harmful. Usually we can see redness, swelling and fever in an area or part of the body that is inflamed
9. respiration	i. your heart rate
10. systolic	j. an act of inhaling and exhaling; a breath

Vital Signs

Vital signs include the measurement of temperature, respiratory rate, pulse, and blood pressure. These numbers provide critical information (hence the name "vital") about a patient's state of health. In particular, they can identify the existence of an acute medical problem.

The more deranged the vitals, the sicker the patient. [1]

Many factors such as sleep, eating, weather, noise, exercise, medications, fear, anxiety, and illness, may cause vital signs to change, sometimes beyond the normal range.

1. Temperature

Temperature is generally obtained using an oral thermometer that provides a digital reading when the sensor is placed under the patient's tongue. So we have oral temperature. The other two common places to take temperature are the rectum and the axilla.

Temperature can be measured by two scales: either in Fahrenheit (F) or Celsius (C) degrees. [2] The average normal adult oral temperature is 98.6℉ (37℃); the rectal temperature 99.6℉ (37.5℃); and the axillary temperature 98℉ (36.7℃).

Many factors, such as age, infection, temperature of the environment, amount of exercise, and emotional status, can affect a patient's temperature and should be considered when a temperature reading is evaluated. For example, the lowest temperature occurs between about 2 a.m. and 6 a.m., and the highest between about 4 p.m. and 8 p.m.

Selection of the appropriate method for obtaining the body temperature depends on several factors, such as age, consciousness level, and emotional status of the patient. For example, the oral method is contraindicated for a small child, a confused or unconscious patient, or patients with pain, injury, or inflammation of the mouth.

2. Respiratory Rate

Respiration is defined as the process of inhaling oxygen-bearing air into the lungs and exhaling carbon dioxide out of the lungs. When a person inhales, his chest expands. When he exhales, his chest contracts.

Respirations are recorded as breaths per minute. Normal respiration rates for an adult at rest range from 16 to 20 breaths per minute. While you are counting respirations, try to do it as surreptitiously as possible so that the patient does not consciously alter their rate of breathing. A good way is remaining your fingers on the patient's wrist after the pulse has been taken and counting the rise and fall of his chest for 30 seconds, then multiplying by 2 and recording.③ During this procedure, a watch displaying seconds④ is needed.

There are different terms used to describe the characteristics of respirations. For example, the patient having difficulty in breathing is said to have dyspnea. Apnea describes the absence of respiration. Rapid respiration is termed tachypnea.

3. Pulse

Your pulse is your heart rate, or the number of times your heart beats in one minute. The quality and rhythm of the pulse must also be observed and described. The normal pulse rhythm is regular, with a steady length of time between each beat.⑤ Normal is between 60 and 100.

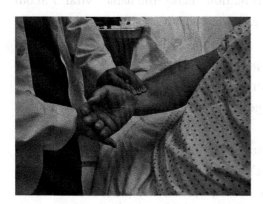

Pulse can be measured at any place where there is a large artery (e. g., carotid, femoral, or simply by listening over the heart), though for the sake of convenience it is generally done by taking the pulse at the radial artery of the wrist. Push lightly at first, adding pressure if there is a lot of subcutaneous fat or you are unable to detect a pulse. If you push too hard, you might occlude the vessel and mistake your own pulse for that of the patient.⑥

4. Blood Pressure

Blood pressure is a measurement of the force applied to the walls of the arteries as the heart pumps blood through the body.⑦

There are two readings when you measure blood pressure, the higher one is called the systolic blood pressure (SBP) and the lower one the diastolic blood pressure (DBP). Normal blood pressure ranges from 100 to 140 millimeters (as the heart beats) over 60 to 90 millimeters (as the heart relaxes). Blood pressure is usually written, for example, as 120/80 mmHg. Normal is between 100/60 and 140/90. Hypertension is thus defined as either SBP greater then 140 or DBP greater than 90. A systolic blood pressure below 100 is termed hypotension, which may not require medical treatment.

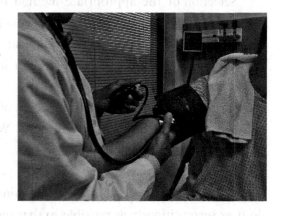

Variations in blood pressure can be caused by several factors, such as age, exercise, emotion, and pain.

To measure the blood pressure, you need a

cuff and a sphygmomanometer. Try to use them appropriately; otherwise the accuracy of these readings will be affected.

Words and Expressions

acute/əˈkjuːt/*adj*.严重的,〈医〉急性的;敏锐的;激烈的

medication/ˌmedɪˈkeʃən/*n*.药物;药物治疗;药物处理

digital/ˈdɪdʒɪtl/*adj*.数字的;手指的

rectum/ˈrektəm/*n*.直肠

contraindicate/ˌkɒntrəˈɪndəˌkeɪt/*vt*.禁忌(某种疗法或药物);显示(治疗或处置)不当

surreptitious/ˌsʌrəpˈtɪʃəs/*adj*.秘密的;鬼鬼祟祟的;暗中的

multiply/ˈmʌltɪplaɪ/*vt*.乘;使增加;使繁殖;使相乘

subcutaneous/ˌsʌbkjuˈteɪnɪəs/*adj*.皮下的;皮下用的

occlude/əˈkluːd/*vt*.使闭塞;封闭;挡住

hypotension/haɪpəʊˈtenʃən/*n*.低血压,血压过低

sphygmomanometer/sfɪɡməʊməˈnɒmɪtə/*n*.〈内科〉血压计

Notes

① "the＋比较级＋(主＋谓),the＋比较级＋(主＋谓)"意为"越……越……",表示一方的程度随着另一方的变化而变化。在通常情况下,如果主、从句中的谓语动词是联系动词 be,且主语为非代词时,此时 be 常常省略。e.g. The higher the tree (is), the stronger the wind (is).树大招风。

② 温度的测算标准有两种:华氏和摄氏。在我国,习惯于以摄氏测算温度。

③ 正确方法是在你测完脉搏后仍然把手放在病人的手腕上,数病人的胸部起伏次数 30 秒,然后乘以 2,再做记录。

④ 秒表。

⑤ 正常脉率跳动均匀规律,间隔时间相等。

⑥ 如果按压腕动脉过度,会使血管闭塞而导致测出的脉率不准。

⑦ 血压是心脏喷射的血液在动脉血管壁上所呈现出来的压力。

Text Exploration

Decide whether the following sentence is true or false. If it is true, put "T" in the bracket, if it is false, put "F" in the bracket.

1. Vital signs include three measures for a person: temperature, pulse and blood pressure. (   )

2. The temperature of an unconscious patient can be measured by placing the sensor under his tongue. (   )

3. Apnea, is the feeling that one cannot breathe well enough or he is short of breath. (   )

4. Normal heart beats in one minute is between 60 and 100. (   )

5. A systolic blood pressure below 100 is termed hypotension，which may not require medical treatment. （　　）

Part II Dialogue ··

Read the following dialogue. Then do Role-play task by using the Sentence Models with your partner.

（A nurse is going to check a patient's vital signs in a medical ward.）

Nurse：Good morning. Ms. Zhang. My name is Wang Mei，your nurse. How are you doing today?

Patient：Good morning. I feel better today.

Nurse：That's good. I'll be checking your vital signs.

Patient：All right.

Nurse：Within the last 30 minutes，have you done any strenuous exercise? Have you had any cold or hot food or drinks? Have you taken a shower?

Patient：No. I've just had my breakfast 40 minutes ago.

Nurse：That's great! Let's begin by checking your temperature. Please put the thermometer under your arm.

Patient：How long should I leave it under my arm?

Nurse：About 10 minutes. Now please give me your wrist. I will also take your pulse and breathing.

（Ten minutes later.）

Patient：How is my temperature，pulse and breathing?

Nurse：Your temperature is 36.5℃，pulse 90 and respiration 20. All are OK with you.

Patient：Good. Thank you.

Nurse：My pleasure. I still need to take your blood pressure. Would you mind rolling up your sleeve and lifting your arm a little so I can put on the cuff?

Patient：No problem.

Nurse：It will feel a little tight on your arm for a few seconds. Please relax.

（After a few seconds.）

Nurse：Your blood pressure is 120/85. Let me help you roll down your sleeve.

Patient：Is it normal?

Nurse：It's within the normal range. Your vitals look pretty good. Alright，we are all done.

Patient：I'm so glad to hear that.

Nurse：Here is the call button. If you need anything else，press the button and I will be back to check. Have a nice day!

Patient：All right. Thank you，Wang Mei.

Nurse：You are welcome.

Words and Expressions

strenuous/ˈstrenjʊəs/ *adj*. 紧张的；费力的；奋发的

thermometer/θəˈmɒmɪtə/ *n*. 温度计；体温计

respiration/ˌrespəˈreɪʃən/ *n*. 呼吸；呼吸作用

roll up 卷起，上滚

sleeve/sliːv/ *n*. [机]套管，[服装]袖套

cuff/kʌf/ *n*. 袖带

Sentence Models

I'll be checking your vital signs.

Within the last 30 minutes, have you done any strenuous exercise? Have you had any cold or hot food or drinks? Have you taken a shower?

Please put the thermometer under your arm.

Now please give me your wrist. I will also take your pulse and breathing.

I still need to take your blood pressure.

Would you mind rolling up your sleeve and lifting your arm a little so I can put on the cuff?

It will feel a little tight on your arm for a few seconds. Please relax.

Let me help you roll down your sleeve.

Your vitals look pretty good.

Role-play

Make a dialogue. Student A acts as a patient; student B acts as a nurse who is going to take BP for the patient.

Use the the above Sentence Models as guidelines.

Part Ⅲ Scene Practice ···

Taking Blood Pressure

Purpose：to observe patient's SBP and DBP to assist diagnosis and treatment.

Preparing

1. Nurse：Wear the uniform, nurse's cap, shoes and mask. Wash your hands.

2. Patient：Explain the procedure of the patient. Let patient understand the notes of the procedure and make ready for it.

3. Equipment：A stethoscope and sphygmomanometer, paper and a pen.

4. Environment：A neat and quiet ward.

Standards and Procedures

Action	Nursing Expressions
1. Gather equipment. Check the bed card. Ask the patient about activities (generally require the patient to have a 5 to 10 min break) 2. Select blood pressure measurement site (e. g., test BP on brachial artery)	—Hello, Mrs. Zhou. I'm going to take your blood pressure.
3. Have the patient assume a comfortable lying or sitting position with the forearm supported at the level of the heart and the palm of the hand upward	—Lie down on the couch and relax, please.
4. Expose the area of the brachial artery by removing garments, or move a sleeve. If it is not too tight, above the area where the cuff will be placed	—Now, please expose your upper arm and the palms facing upwards.
5. Center the bladder of the cuff over the brachial approximately midway on the arm, so that the lower edge of the cuff is about 2 to 3 cm above the inner aspect of the elbow. The tubing should extend from the edge of the cuff nearer the patient's elbow	
6. Wrap the cuff around the arm smoothly and snugly, and fasten it securely or tuck the end of the cuff well under the preceding wrapping	
7. Tighten the screw valve on the air pump. Deflate the cuff and wait 15 seconds	
8. Pump the pressure 20 to 30 mmHg (2.7 to 4 kPa) above the point at which the pulse disappeared. Open the valve on the manometer and allow air to escape slowly so that the pressure decrease at the rate of 4 mmhg per second. Notice scales on the mercury tube and the changes of voice of brachial artery. The first voice of the brachial pulse heard is systolic pressure and the hanged voice or disappearance of the brachial pulse heard is diastolic pressure	—If you feel discomfortable, please let me know.
9. Expel the air of the cuff to set the mercury down to zero before re-measure the blood pressure. Wait a moment and start the second measure. Get the mini-value from 2 to 3 continuous measurement	
10. Expel the air of the cuff after having taken BP and make the lid of the sphygmomanometer toward 45 degree so that all mercury of the glass tube return to the mercury tank, close the mercury switch device, lay the upper lid and replace flatly the sphygmomanometer	
11. Arrange linens on the bed in order, remove all equipment 12. Wash your hands and record the values of BP	—Thanks for your cooperation. Your BP is 120/80. It is within the normal range. If you need any help, please press the button. Have a good rest.

Words and Expressions

bladder/ˈblædə/ *n*. 膀胱;囊状物

snugly/ˈsnʌɡlɪ/*adv*. 紧贴地;贴身地;暖和舒适地

valve/vælv/*n*. 阀;真空管;(管乐器的)活栓;(心脏的)瓣膜

deflate/dɪˈflet/*v*. 放气;瘪下来;使泄气;紧缩

manometer/məˈnɒmətə/*n*. 压力计

lid/lɪd/*n*. 盖子;限制

Critical Thinking

Work in pairs and discuss the following questions.

1. Explain the necessity of removing the patient's sleeve when putting on the cuff.

2. How would you distinguish the different voices of brachial artery between systolic pressure and diastolic pressure by using stethoscope?

3. What's the purpose of allowing air in the manometer to escape slowly and thus keeping pressure decrease at the rate of 4 mmHg per second?

4. If you get an abnormal result of the patient after taking his BP for once, what you are going to do?

Unit 4

Routes of Administration

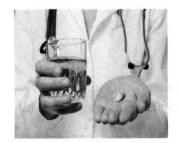 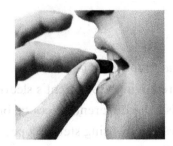 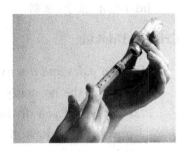

Part I **Text** ....

Warming-up

1. How many common routes of administration do you know?
2. Can you describe one of the routes of administration in detail?

Topic-related Terms

Match the words Column A with their meanings in Column B.

Column A	Column B
1. optic	a. the act of giving a drug to somebody
2. parenteral	b. toward the inside of the cheek
3. intradermal	c. areas located below the epidermis
4. administration	d. relating to the ear
5. buccal	e. tissue under skin
6. subcutaneous	f. the surface of a body part
7. topical	g. relating to or resembling the eye
8. otic	h. administered by means other than through the alimentary tract

The Routes of Administration

A route of administration in pharmacology and toxicology is the path by which a drug, fluid, poison, or other substance is taken into the body. Routes of administration are generally classified by the location at which the substance is applied. Common examples include oral and intravenous administration. Routes can also be classified based on where the target of action is. Action may be topical (local), enteral (system-wide effect, but delivered through the gastrointestinal tract), or parenteral (systemic action, but delivered by routes other than the GI tract).

Medications are administered in different ways:

A. Oral is the most common method, i. e. given by mouth. Any medication given by mouth may be considered an oral medication. Even if the absorption of drugs begins in the mouth, most of them are absorbed in the stomach or intestines. It can be classified into:

1. Sublingual medications: agents placed under the tongue and absorbed into the blood vessels underneath the tongue.

2. Buccal medications: medication held inside the mouth against the mucous membrane of the cheek. Buccal tablets are often harder tablets (4 hours disintegration time), designed to dissolve slowly.

The advantages of oral medication including:

- First pass—The liver is by-passed. Thus there is no loss of drug by first pass effect for buccal administration. Bioavailability is higher.
- Rapid absorption—Because of the good blood supply to the area, absorption is usually quite rapid.
- Drug stability—pH in mouth relatively is neutral (cf. stomach-acidic). Thus a drug may be more stable.

B. Nasogastric administration routes:

    1. Indications:

        1) normal gastric emptying

        2) stomach uninvolved with primary disease

    2. Advantages:

        1) easy tube insertion

        2) intact gag reflex

        3) no esophageal reflux

        4) larger reservoir capacity in stomach

C. Topical medications: agents applied to the skin and mucous membranes for absorption or for local therapy. In addition to administration onto the skin, topical agents include:

    1. optic medications (medications administered into the eye);

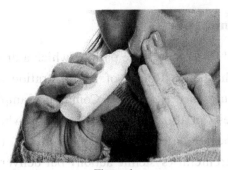

Figure 1

2. otic medications（medications administered into the ear）;

3. nasal medications（medications administered into the nose）(See Figure 1);

4. vaginal medications（medications administered into the vagina）;

5. rectal medications（medications inserted or instilled into the rectum）;

6. pulmonary medications（medications inhaled into the respiratory tract）.

D. Parenteral medications: given by injection with a needle. Parenteral medications are the most rapidly absorbed because they are administered directly into or close to the circulation. Routes of administration for parenteral medications include:

1. subcutaneous (SC) route: administration into the subcutaneous tissue, under the skin;

2. intravenous (IV) route: administration into a vein;

3. intramuscular (IM) route: administration into a muscle (See Figure 2);

4. intradermal (ID) route: administration into the epidermis, into the dermis;

5. intra-arterial (IA)route: administration into an artery;

6. intracardiac route: administration into the heart muscle;

7. intraosseous route: administration into a bone;

8. intrathecal route: administration into the spinal canal;

9. epidural route: administration into the space external to the duramater of the spinal canal(See Figure 3).

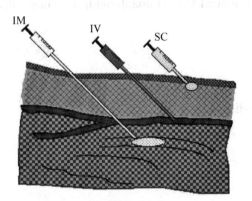

Figure 2

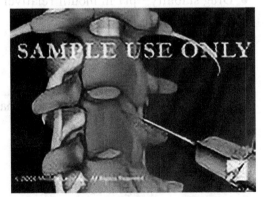

Figure 3

Words and Expressions

administration/ədˌmɪnɪsˈtreɪʃən/ n . 给药,管理,实施

intestine/ɪnˈtestɪn/ n . 肠内

sublingual/sʌbˈlɪŋgwəl/*adj.*舌下的

mucous/ˈmjuːkəs/*adj.*黏液的

membrane/ˈmemˌbreɪn/*n.*薄膜，隔膜

nasogastric/ˌneɪzəʊˈgæstrɪk/*adj.*鼻饲的

esophageal/iːˌsɒfəˈdʒiːəl/*adj.*食道的，食管的

reflux/ˈriːflʌks/*n.*逆流，反流

gastric/ˈgæstrɪk/*adj.*胃的，胃部的

reservoir/ˈrezəvwɑː/*n.*蓄积

therapy/ˈθerəpɪ/*n.*治疗，疗法

optic/ˈɒptɪk/*adj.*眼睛的，视觉的

otic/ˈəʊtɪk/*adj.*耳的

nasal/ˈneɪzəl/*adj.*鼻的

vaginal/ˈvædʒənəl/*adj.*阴道的

rectal/ˈrekt(ə)l/*adj.*直肠的

pulmonary/ˈpʊlməˌnerɪ/*adj.*肺的，肺部的

parenteral/pæˈrentərəl/*adj.*肠胃外的

subcutaneous/ˌsʌbkjuːˈteɪniːəs/*adj.*皮下的

intradermal/ˌɪntrəˈdəːml/*adj.*皮内的，皮层内的

intramuscular/ˌɪntrəˈmʌskjʊlə/*adj.*肌肉的

intravenous/ˌɪntrəˈviːnəs/*adj.*静脉注射的

intracardiac/ˌɪntrəˈkɑːdɪæk/*adj.*心脏内的

intraosseous/ɪntˈrəɒsɪəs/*adj.*骨内的

intrathecal/ˌɪntrəˈθiːkəl/*adj.*鞘内的，膜内的

epidural/ˌepɪˈdjʊərəl/*adj.*硬(脑)膜上的

Text Exploration

Decide whether the following sentence is true or false. If it is true, put "T" in the bracket, if it is false, put "F" in the bracket.

1. Agents placed under the tongue and absorbed into the blood vessels underneath the tongue are called sublingual medications. (   )
2. Nasal medications refer to medications administered into the nose. (   )
3. Intravenous (IV) route means administration into a muscle. (   )
4. Intra-arterial (IA) route means administration into the heart muscle. (   )
5. Pulmonary medications refer to medications inhaled into the respiratory tract. (   )

Part Ⅱ Dialogue ....

Read the following dialogue. Then do the Role-Play task by using the Sentence Models with your partner.

Starting an IV

Nurse: Good morning. Are you Mrs. Zhang, bed 38? It is time for me to give you IV fluids.

Patient: What is an IV?

Nurse: It is a small plastic needle that is inserted into a vein. The fluid in the bottle goes into your body through the tubing and needle.

Patient: What is in the bottle?

Nurse: It is sugar and water. You are not able to eat after the operation, so this is your food.

Patient: Will it hurt?

Nurse: Don't worry. Just take it easy. When I put it in, it might be a little uncomfortable, but after that it won't hurt.

(The nurse puts on a tourniquet and looks for a good vein in Mrs. Zhang's left hand.)

Nurse: Please make a fist, I have found a spot. Okay, you will feel a prick. Please try not to move until I tell you. It is in. I am turning on the IV. Please don't move yet. I need to tape it securely. All right, you can move now. Remember to keep your arm lower than your heart. The IV should drip at this speed. Do not change the flow rate by yourself.

Patient: Why don't you let the fluid run more quickly?

Nurse: Your IV fluids must be given slowly so as not to overload you. If you feel any pain or burning at this site, or if you see any welling or redness, please let us know as soon as possible. I will be back soon to check if the blood backs up or the bottle is empty.

Words and Expressions

insert/ɪn'sət/ vt. 插入；嵌入
vein/veɪn/ n. 静脉
tourniquet/'tʊrnɪkɪt/ n. 止血带
fist/fɪst/ n. 拳头
prick/prɪk/ n. 扎，刺

Sentence Model

1. It is time for me to give you IV fluids.
2. Please make a fist, I have found a spot.
3. Please try not to move until I tell you.
4. I am going to clean the area with betadine and then alcohol.
5. I need to tape it securely.
6. Remember to keep your arm lower than your heart.
7. Your IV fluids must be given slowly so as not to overload you.

Role-play

Student A acts a nurse, and student B acts a patient. Make a dialogue on oral administration. The following information may serve as guidelines.

Medicines	Time	Dose
a glass bottle of white tablets	after meals	1 tablet 3 times a day
a plastic bottle of red pills	morning and evening	2 tablets twice a day
cough syrup(咳嗽糖浆)	when needed	not more than 6 tablespoonful a day

Part Ⅲ Scene Practice

The Allergic Test to Penicillin

Purpose：To test body's allergies to penicillin.

Preparing

1. **Nurse** Wear the uniform, nurse's cap, shoes and mask. File nails short and wash your hands.

2. **Patient** Explain the aims and guidelines of administering intradermal injection to the patient.

3. **Equipment** One milliliter sterile syringe, 5 milliliters sterile syringe, sterile container and sterile forceps, sterile swabs, 75% alcohol, iodophor, penicillin (800,000U), kidney basin, sterile gauze, sterile normal saline, abrasive, sterile package, box for first aid including 2 epinephrine, 1 dxamethasone, abrasive, sterile gauze, two sterile syringes (2 to 5 milliliters), bottle-opener.

4. **Environment** The environment should be clean, spacious and bright.

Standards and Procedures

Action	Nursing Expression
(1) Check the doctor's order, apply the sterile treatment tray. (2) Dilute the solution for skin test. ① Cleanse the vial-neck and metal file with iodophor; scratch the vial neck and cleanse it with the alcohol; and then break it off. ② Aspirate 4 ml of normal saline and then insert the needle into the vial of penicillin and dissolve it completely. ③ Aspirate 0.1 ml of the dissolved solution and add 0.9 ml of normal saline with a set of 1 ml syringe and then shake well; discard 0.9 ml of solution, add 0.9 ml of normal saline and then shake well; discard 0.9 ml or 0.75 ml of solution again, add 0.9 ml or 0.75 ml of normal saline and then shake well.	—Hello! Liu Li, have you had breakfast? Now I want to give you a skin test.

（续表）

④ Change a new needle; protect the needle from contamination with a plastic cap and then put it in a sterile treatment tray. (3) Arrange a set of equipment on a tray in order of use and carry it to the patient's bedside, explain the aims of injection to the patient, recheck the medical history, allergic history and family history after reading the bed card of the patient.	
(4) Assist patients to take a comfortable posture, roll up sleeves to elbow, selected the injection site (one-third under the inner bone of the forearm), cleanse the injection site with 75% alcohol (avoid disinfectants with iodine, alcohol allergies with a saline solution to wipe clean the skin), expel air bubbles and recheck.	—Please relax and don't be nervous. Let me help you roll up your sleeves.
(5) Grasp the forearm to be injected with the left hand. Insert the needle, with the bevel of the needle facing upward, insert the needle under the outer layer of the skin at an angle almost parallel to the skin (0 to 5 degree), insert the needle so that only the bevel penetrates the skin and inject 0.1 ml of the solution slowly. If you have inserted the needle correctly, a small circular bubble of the solution forms just under the thin outer layer of the skin.	
(6) Withdraw the needle quickly. (7) Inform patient the attention. (8) Check it again; remove the equipment, tidy up the bed unit.	—Do you have any discomfort? I will see the result 20 minutes later, in the meantime, please do not leave the ward, never press or scratch the injection site. If you feel discomfort please tell us in time.
(9) Twenty minutes later, observe the results (negative response: the small circular bubble has no change; the tissue around the bubble is in the absence of the rubefaction, pseudopod, and itch, the patient has no uncomfortable feeling. Positive response: the diameter of the small circular bubble is beyond to 1cm; the tissue around the bubble is in the presence of the rubefaction, pseudopod, and itch; the patient feels stuffy and dizzy; even anaphylactic shock takes place.)	—Liu Li, do you feel alright? Is anything wrong? Let me see the result, your skin rest was negative. We will give you a penicillin shot.
(10) Record (negative "-" and positive "+"), if positive, give a clear explanation to the patients and families, make an obvious record in transfusion card, the doctor's order, display board, bedside card, and medical card.	

Words and Expressions

saline/ˈseɪˌlɪn/ n. 盐水

syringe/səˈrɪndʒ/ n. 注射器

forceps/ˈfɔrsəps/ n. 镊子

epinephrine/ˌepəˈnefrɪn/ n. 肾上腺素

dxamethasone/ˌdeksəˈmeəˌzəʊn/ n. /药/地塞米松;氟美松（抗炎药）

iodophor/aɪˈəʊdəˌfɔr/ n. 碘伏

aspirate/ˈæspəˌreɪt/ v. 抽出,抽取

sterile/ˈsterəl/ adj. 无菌的

disinfectant/ˌdɪsənˈfektənt/ *n.* 消毒剂；杀菌剂

adj. 消毒的，无菌的

anaphylactic/ˌænəfɪˈlæktɪk/ *adj.* 过敏的

Critical Thinking

Work in pairs and discuss the following questions.

1. What is the purpose of penicillin skin test?
2. What are the symptoms of penicillin allergy?
3. What are treatments of penicillin allergy?
4. What are your options when you are allergic?

Unit 5

Medical Nursing

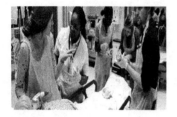 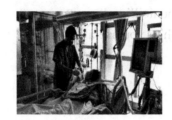 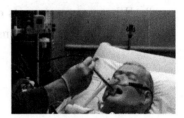

Warming-up

1. Is adequate nutrition necessary for the patient's recovery?
2. If the patient is unable to use the oral route to take sufficient nutrients to maintain growth and development, what is the method to be taken?
3. What's the risk associated with aspiration?

Topic-related Terms

Match the words in Column A with their meanings in Column B.

Column A	Column B
1. nutritional	a. of or relating to the enteron
2. insert	b. the part of the small intestine between the stomach and the jejunum
3. enteral	c. of or relating to or used in or practicing neurology
4. carbohydrate	d. of or relating to or providing nutrition
5. duodenum	e. pour or rush back
6. gastrointestinal	f. simple sugars with small molecules as well as macromolecular substances
7. neurological	g. put or introduce into something
8. regurgitate	h. of or relating to the stomach and intestines

Enteral Feeding

Patients need adequate nutrition to recover from any illness. Patients who are critically ill have high nutritional requirements and can become malnourished very quickly. We know from research findings that early feeding is important to patient outcome. The nutritional needs of all patients are reviewed daily and feeding is initiated as soon as possible, usually within the first day of admission. Enteral 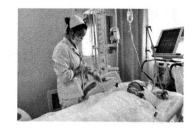 feeding refers to the delivery of a nutritionally complete feed, containing protein, carbohydrate, fat, water, minerals and vitamins, directly into the stomach, duodenum or jejunum.

The best way to feed a patient is using their own gastrointestinal tract (stomach and bowel). Feeding by the gastrointestinal tract is called "enteral feeding". We also refer to this as feeding through the gut. While patients cannot swallow food if they have a breathing tube in their throat, they are fed through a feeding tube. A specially designed solution that contains the nutrients the patient will need to recover is provided.

Gastroenteric tube feeding plays a major role in the management of patients with poor voluntary intake, chronic neurological or mechanical dysphagia or gut dysfunction and in patients who are critically ill. Most feeding tubes are inserted into the nose or the mouth, and the tube is advanced into the stomach. The feeds are mixed in a sterile bag and given as a steady infusion that runs 24 hours per day. A pump similar to an intravenous pump is used to deliver the feeding solution.

Words and Expressions

adequate/ˈædɪkwət/ adj. 足够的；适当的；能胜任的
nutrition/njʊˈtrɪʃən/ n. 营养
critically/ˈkrɪtɪklɪ/ adv. 批评性地；爱挑剔地；重要地；危急地
malnourished/ˌmælˈnʌrɪʃt/ adj. 营养不良的
outcome/ˈaʊtkʌm/ n. 结果；后果
nutritional/njʊˈtrɪʃənl/ adj. 营养的；滋养的
carbohydrate/ˌkɑːbəʊˈhaɪdreɪt/ n. 碳水化合物；糖类
duodenum/ˌdjuːəˈdiːnəm/ n. 十二指肠
neurological/ˌnjʊərəˈlɒdʒɪkl/ adj. 神经病学的
enteral/ˈentərəl/ adj. 肠的
jejunum/dʒɪˈdʒuːnəm/ n. [解]空肠
dysphagia/dɪsˈfeɪdʒɪə/ n. 吞咽困难
dysfunction/dɪsˈfʌŋkʃn/ n. 功能不良；机能障碍
inserted/ɪnˈsɜːtɪd/ adj. 插入的；嵌入的；着生的；附着的

infusion/ɪnˈfjuːʒn/ *n*. 注入;灌输;激励;泡制

intravenous/ˌɪntrəˈviːnəs/ *adj*. 静脉的;静脉注射的

pump/pʌmp/ *n*. 泵;抽水机;打气筒;抽水;打气

　　　　　 v. 打气;唧筒般运动;灌输;抽取;增加;盘问

gut/ɡʌt/ *n*. 勇气;内脏;直觉;肠

　　　　 adj. 本能的,直觉的

　　　　 vt. 毁坏(建筑物等)的内部;取出……的内脏

Notes

被动语态

用法：不知道动作的执行者是谁;动作的承受者是谈话的中心。

结构：助动词 be＋动词的过去分词

　　　　一般现在时：am/is/are＋过去分词

　　　　一般过去时：was/were＋过去分词

　　　　一般将来时：will/shall＋be＋过去分词

　　　　现在完成时：has/have＋been＋过去分词

　　　　过去完成时：had＋been＋过去分词

　　　　过去将来时：would/should＋be＋过去分词

　　　　现在进行时：am/is/are＋being＋过去分词

　　　　过去进行时：was/were＋being＋过去分词

　　　　含情态动词的被动语态：情态动词＋be＋过去分词

Text Exploration

Decide whether the following sentence is true or false. If it is true, put "T" in the bracket, if it is false, put "F" in the bracket.

1. "Enteral feeding" also refers to feeding through the gut. （　　）

2. The enteral feeding is reviewed daily within the first day of admission. （　　）

3. The best way to feed a patient is using tubes inserted into the nose or the mouth, and the tube is advanced into the stomach. （　　）

4. Enteral feeding means to the delivery of nutrition. （　　）

5. Gastroenteric tube feeding plays a major role in the management of the critically ill. （　　）

Part Ⅱ　Dialogue ....

Read the following dialogue. Then do Role-play task by using the Sentence Models with your partner.

Doctor：What seems to be the problem?

Patient：I got indigestion.

Doctor：How does the indigestion affect you?

Patient：All the food stays up here(indicating chest).

Doctor：When do you get it?

Patient：Two to three hours after food.

Doctor：What is it like? A pain?

Patient：Yes, a pain.

Doctor：What kind? Burning, stabbing?

Patient：It feels like some wind there and I want to get rid of it.

Doctor：Do you belch?

Patient：Not much.

Doctor：Does it bother you at night?

Patient：No.

Doctor：It comes on when you are hungry?

Patient：Yes, I have a terrible pain in my stomach and I feel I'll collapse if I don't eat straight away.

Doctor：How is your appetite?

Patient：Very poor.

Doctor：Did you always have a bad one?

Patient：No, it started to deteriorate ten years ago.

Doctor：Has it changed much in the last few months?

Patient：I think the medicine must push the food down and then I fell hungry.

Doctor：You'd better take some tests. I will prescribe some for you after taking tested.

Patient：Any instructions I should be paying special attention to?

Doctor：Don't eat anything cold or spicy.

Words and Expressions

indigestion/ˌɪndɪˈdʒestʃən/n.消化不良

burning/ˈbɜːnɪŋ/adj.燃烧的

stabbing/ˈstæbɪŋ/adj.刺痛的

belch/beltʃ/v.打嗝

collapse/kəˈlæps/v.(使)崩溃

deteriorate/dɪˈtɪərɪəreɪt/v.恶化

instruction/ɪnˈstrʌkʃən/n.指令;教学;教诲;说明

Sentence Models

What seems to be the problem?

When do you get it?

You'd better take some tests. I will prescribe some for you after taking tested.

Any instructions I should be paying special attention to?

Role-play

Make a dialogue. Student A acts as a patient who is seeing a doctor acted by Student B for some kinds of disease.

Use the above Sentence Models as guidelines.

Part Ⅲ Scene Practice ....

Read the information below about the procedure of nasogastric intubation. Make sure about the correct ways and procedures of nasogastric intubation.

Purpose: to master the procedure of nasogastric intubation.

Preparing:

1. Nurse: Gathering together all the equipment needed and place on a clean tray. Wash and dry hands thoroughly, put on non-sterile gloves and apron.

2. Equipment: The appropriate size and type of tube, sterile water, foil bowl and tissues, pH indicator paper, 20 ml syringe, non-sterile gloves, tape.

3. Environment: A neat and quiet ward.

Standards and Procedures:

1. Find the most appropriate position for the patient, depending on age and ability to co-operate. Ensure the chosen nostril is clear of debris. Ask the patient, if age appropriate, which side they would prefer to have the tube positioned.

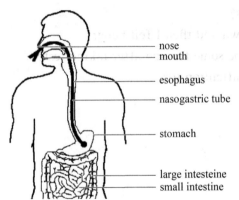

nose
mouth

esophagus

nasogastric tube

stomach

large intesteine
small intestine

2. a. Check that the tube is intact. The tube should be stretched to remove any shape retained from being packaged. If the tube has a guide wire, make sure it is correctly inserted in the tube and is not bent. If the tube has a guide wire, it is helpful to flush the tube with 10 ml of sterile water before insertion.

b. For infants and children: measure the length of tube to be inserted. Measure from the bridge of the nose to the ear lobe, then from the ear lobe to xiphisternum. The length of tube can be marked with indelible pen or a note taken of the measurement marks on the tube.

c. For neonates: measure from the nose to ear and then to the halfway point between xiphisternum and umbilicus.

d. Lubricate the end of the tube in sterile water; do not use K-Y Jelly.

e. Bend the patient's head slightly forward and gently pass the tube into the patient's nostril, advancing it along the floor of the nasopharynx to the oropharynx. At this point, ask the patient to swallow a little water or offer a younger child their soother, to assist passage of the tube down the oesophagus until the required length of tube has been inserted.

f. Never advance the tube against resistance. If the patient shows signs of breathlessness or severe coughing, remove the tube immediately.

g. Lightly secure the tube with tape, or have an assistant hold the tube in place until the position has been checked.

Words and Expressions

nostril/ˈnɒstrəl/ n. 鼻孔

debris/ˈdebriː/ n. 碎片；残骸

intact/ɪnˈtækt/ adj. 完好无缺的；原封不动的；未经触碰的

guide wire 尺度索，准绳

flush/flʌʃ/ v. 冲洗；发红；将某人赶出　n. 脸红；冲洗；(纸牌)同花牌

sterile/ˈsteraɪl/ adj. 贫瘠的；无生气的；无生育能力的；无结果的；无菌的

xiphisternum/ˌzɪfɪˈstɜːnəm/ n. [解][动]剑胸骨

neonates/ˈniːəʊneɪt/ n. [哺乳动物]新生儿

umbilicus/ʌmˈbɪlɪkəs/ n. [生]脐；[植]种脐；中心；核心

lubricate/ˈluːbrɪkeɪt/ v. 润滑；加润滑剂

nasopharynx/ˌneɪzəʊˈfærɪŋks/ n. 鼻咽

oropharynx/əʊrəˈfærɪŋks/ n. [解]口咽

soother/ˈsuːðə(r)/ n. 抚慰者；安神物

oesophagus/ɪˈsɒfəgəs/ n. 食道

Critical Thinking

Work in pairs and discuss the following questions.

1. What procedures do you think should be included in the nasogastric intubation?
2. What preparation should be done before the nasogastric intubation?
3. What determine the most appropriate position of nasogastric intubation?
4. What should be done when being against resistance?

Unit 6

Surgical Nursing

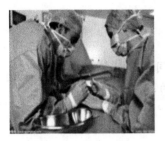 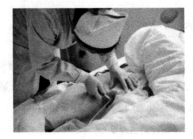 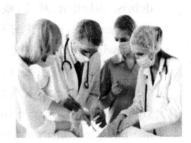

Part I Text

Warming-up

1. What does healthy care include today?
2. What are the roles of medical-surgical nurses?
3. What does a medical nurse usually do as a caregiver?

Topic-related Terms

Match the words in Column A with their meanings in Column B.

Column A	Column B
1. caregiver	a. the act of taking action that has been officially decided to happen
2. assessment	b. someone who takes care of a child or sick person
3. implementation	c. a doctor, especially one who is a specialist in general medicine and not surgery
4. physician	d. the service of providing medical care
5. healthcare	e. the act of judging or forming an opinion about sb. /sth.

Roles of the Nurse in Medical-surgical Nursing Practice

Health care today is a vast and complex system. It reflects changes in society, changes in

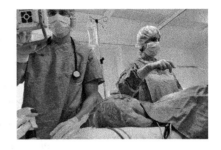

the populations requiring nursing care, and a philosophical shift toward health promotion rather than illness care. The roles of the medical-surgical nurse have broadened and expanded in response to these changes. Medical-surgical nurses are caregivers but also educators, advocates, leaders and managers, and researchers.① The nurse assumes these various roles to promote and maintain health, to prevent illness, and to facilitate coping with disability or death for the adult client (a person requiring healthcare services) in any setting.

Nurses have always been caregivers. However, the activities carried out within the caregiver role have changed tremendously in the 21st century. From 1900 to the 1960s, the nurse was almost always female and was regarded primarily as the person who gave personal care and carried out physician's orders. This dependent role has changed as a result of the increased education of nurses, research in and the development of nursing knowledge and the recognition that nurses are autonomous and informed professionals.

The caregiver role for the nurse today is both independent and collaborative. Nurses independently make assessments and plan and implement client care based on nursing knowledge and skills. Nurses also collaborate with other members of the healthcare team to complement and evaluate care.

As a caregiver, the nurse is practitioner of nursing both as a science and as an art. Using critical thinking in the nursing process as the framework for care, the nurse provides interventions to meet not only the physical needs but also the psychosocial, cultural, spiritual, and environmental needs of clients and families.② Considering all aspects of the client ensures a holistic approach to nursing. Holistic nursing care is based on a philosophical view that interacting wholes are greater than the sum of their parts. A holistic approach also emphasizes the uniqueness of the individual.

In providing comprehensive, individualized care, the nurse uses critical thinking skills to analyze and synthesize knowledge from the arts, the sciences, and nursing research and theory. The science of nursing is translated into the art of nursing through caring. Caring is the means by which the nurse is connected with and concerned for the client. Thus, the nurse as caregiver is knowledgeable, skilled, empathic, and caring.

Words and Expressions

complex/kəmˈpleks/*adj*.复杂的;难懂的;复合的;

　　　　　　n.情结;建筑群;相关联的一组事物;不正常的忧虑

caregiver/ˈkeɪɡɪvə(r)/*n*.照料者,护理者

philosophical/ˌfɪləˈsɑːfɪkl/*adj*.哲学上的,哲学(家)的;冷静的,沉着的;明达

advocate/ˈædvəˌkeɪt/*vt*.提倡;鼓吹;拥护;为……辩护;

　　　　　　n.提倡者;(辩护)律师;支持者

maintain/meɪnˈteɪn/ *vt*. 保持；保养；坚持

facilitate/fəˈsɪlɪˌteɪt/ *vt*. 帮助；促进，助长；使容易

physician/fɪˈzɪʃən/ *n*. 医生，内科医生；〈口〉医学博士；（精神创伤的）医治者，抚慰者

collaborative/kəˈlæbəreɪtɪv/ *adj*. 协作的；合作的

holistic/həʊˈlɪstɪk/ *adj*. 全盘的，整体的；功能整体性的

synthesize/ˈsɪnθɪˌsaɪz/ *vt*. 综合；人工合成；（通过化学手段或生物过程）合成；（音响）合成；
　　　　　　　　　　 vi. 合成；综合

empathic/emˈpæθɪk/ *adj*. 感情移入的

Notes

① 护士是教育者、倡导者、领导者、管理者和研究者，而不再仅仅是护理者。

② not only...but also... 不但……而且……

在护理过程中要以批判性思维作为整个护理工作的框架，不再是单纯的疾病护理，而是以"病人及其家属"为中心的心理、文化、精神以及环境等的全方位护理，是考虑到病人各种需求的整体护理。

Text Exploration

Decide whether the following sentence is true or false. If it is true, put "T" in the bracket, if it is false, put "F" in the bracket.

1. Health care today reflects changes in society, in the populations and a philosophical shift toward health promotion rather than illness care. （　　）

2. The roles of the medical-surgical nurse are caregivers, educators, advocates, leaders and managers, and researchers. （　　）

3. The nurse was almost always female and was regarded primarily as the person who gave personal care and carried out physician's orders. （　　）

4. Holistic nursing care is based on a philosophical view that interacting wholes are greater than the sum of their parts. （　　）

5. Caring is the means by which the nurse is connected with and concerned for the patient. （　　）

Part Ⅱ　Dialogue

Read the following dialogue. Then do Role-play task by using the Sentence Models with your partner.

（In the surgical ward, a nurse is talking to Mr. Li about the instructions of the scheduled operation）

Nurse：Hello, Mr. Li, how are you? Are you exercising? （Mr. Li answered with a nod.） Let me check your drainage bag to make sure the fixed position is right. （Nurse Wu bent over to look at the patent's drainage bag.） Very good! The urine is also pretty clear. Did you drink any water this morning?

Patient: I drank a cup of water this morning, Miss Wu. Could you help me to ask the doctor if he can operate on me as soon as possible?

Nurse: Don't worry, Mr. Li, the operation is set for tomorrow. Yesterday, I told you about the operation procedures and how you can cooperate with us. Do you still have anything unclear that I can help you with?

Patient: I understand them well because I have studied the materials you gave me several times. Let me show you. (Mr. Li began to restate the information about the operation. Nurse Wu listened and made a few corrections from time to time.)

Nurse: Mr. Li, you have a good memory. Now, let us practice relaxing, deep breathing, and effective coughing. Please lie down on the bed first. (Nurse Wu helped him to lie down on the bed and he began to practice.) Close your mouth when you take a deep breath. Use your nose to inhale and relax your hands. Good. Let's try again.

Nurse: Mr. Li, your operation tomorrow will need epidural anesthesia, that is, lower body anesthesia. The anesthetic drug will be injected to your spine and you'll have no feelings in your lower half body after the injection, but you will remain conscious. Now I'll teach you how to cooperate with doctor. Mr. Li, please lie on your side and bend your legs to your chest, use your arms to hold your knees. (Nurse Wu helped Mr. Li to hold his knees with his arms.) Try to make your back protruding and lower your head. Good, that's right. I'm going to care for other patients now. But I'll be back later to do some preoperative preparations for you. Mr. Li, you can sit back and chat with Mr. Zhang on bed 26 who had the similar operation as yours.

(Nurse Wu asked Mr. Zhang to talk to Mr. Li about his operation experience. After completing nursing care on the other patients, Nurse Wu came back and finished Mr. Li's preoperative preparations.)

Words and Expressions

drainage/ˈdreɪnɪdʒ/ n. 排水系统；排水，放水；排走物，废水；排水区域
epidural/ˌepɪˈdʊrəl, -ˈdjʊr-/ adj. 硬(脑)膜上的，硬脑膜外的
anesthesia/ˌænɪsˈθiːʒə/ n. 麻醉；感觉缺失，麻木
spine/spaɪn/ n. 脊柱；脊椎；书脊；(动植物的)刺

Sentence Models

Let me check your drainage bag to make sure the fixed position is right.

I told you about the operation procedures and how you can cooperate with us.

Do you still have anything unclear that I can help you with?

Now I'll teach you how to cooperate with doctor.

Role-play

Make a dialogue. Student A acts as a patient; student B acts as a nurse who is going to talk to the patient before operation.
Do use the Sentence Models as guidelines.

Part Ⅲ Scene Practice

Read the information below about the action of Urinary Catheterization. Make sure about the correct ways and procedures. Student A acts as a patient; student B acts as a nurse and then practise this action with the equipment prepared. Do use the expressions to communicate with each other effectively.

Urinary Catheterization

Purposes

　　1. To empty the bladder to relieve the patent's discomfort.

　　2. To obtain sterile specimen for bacterial culture.

　　3. To assess the amount of residual urine, bladder capacity and bladder pressure to assist in diagnosis.

Preparing

　　1. Nurse: Wear the uniform, nurse's cap, shoes and mask. File nails short and wash your hands.

　　2. Patient: Explain the aim to the patient. Let the patient understand the instruction of the procedure and clean genital and perineal area.

　　3. Equipment: Sterile catheterization kit that contains two straight catheters, two forceps, small cotton balls, cotton balls dipped with lubricant, fenestrated drape, two kidney basins, specimen containers, gauze squares and kidney basin; sterile container and sterile forceps, disposable gloves, sterile forceps, iodophor, kidney basin, waterproof pad, cotton drawsheet, bath blanket, pen, record sheet, bedpan and cover, screen of needed. Assemble equipment and arrange on a nursing cart in the order of their use.

　　4. Environment: Close door, windows and curtains. Regulate the room temperature.

Standards and Procedures

Action	Nursing Expressions
1. Assemble equipment. Check the bed card of the patient. Explain the procedure and its purpose to the patient. 2. Assist the patient to take off the trousers and drape the patient appropriately. 3. Position the patient on his/her back with the knees flexed and legs apart. Expose only genital and perineal area.	—Good morning, Mr./Mrs. Zhou. I will insert a catheter to your bladder, urine will come out through the catheter and then you will feel better. Are you ready for it?

（续表）

4. Clean the genital and perineal area.	—Let me help you take off pants.
（1）Open the sterile disinfection kit on bed using sterile technique. Pour antiseptic solution over cotton balls.	—Now, raise your buttocks please.
（2）Put on disposable gloves. Place a kidney basin near the perineum and the treatment bowl between the patient's thighs.	
Male	
（3）Clean the pubes, penis and scrotum with the cotton balls. First mons pubis and labia majoria. And then separate the labia well with the left hand. Clean the area at and around the meatus with cotton balls moistened with antiseptic. Use each cotton ball once and from the area directly above the meatus down toward the anal area.	—Mr./Mrs. Zhou, I'll clean your genital and perineal area.
Female	
（3）Clean the perineal-genital area with the cotton balls. First mons pubis and labia majoria. And then separate the labia with well with the left hand. Clean the area at and around the meatus with cotton balls moistened with antiseptic. Use each cotton ball once and from the area directly above the meatus down toward the anal area.	—Mr./Mrs. Zhou, I'll clean your genital and perineal area.
（4）Place the kidney basin and the treatment bowl on the lower laver of the cart.	
（5）Open the sterile catheterization kit. Pour antiseptic solution over cotton balls.	
（6）Put on sterile gloves. Place the fenestrated drape with opening catheterization kit over the meatus or the penis to create a sterile field.	
（7）Disinfect the genital and perineal area and insert the catheter.	
a. Check the catheter. Lubricate the catheter. Place a kidney basin near the perineum.	
Male	—Please don't move, I need to put a drape between your legs and keep the area aseptic, OK?
b. Lift the penis with your nondominant hand, which is then considered contaminated. Retract the foreskin. Clean the area at the meatus with a cotton ball held with a forceps. Use a circular motion, moving from the meatus toward the base of the penis for three cleansings.	
Hold the penis with slight upward tension and perpendicular to the patient's body. Insert the tip into the meatus about 20 to 22 cm, until urine flows. Do not use force to introduce the catheter. If the catheter resists entry, ask the patient to breathe deeply and rotate the catheter slightly. Insert the catheter in the direction of the urethra. Then insert the catheter 1 to 2 cm more.	—I will sterile your private part, it may be a little bit cold, take it easy.
Female	—Now, please relax and take a deep breath slowly, I will insert the catheter.
b. Using the nondominant hand, separate the labia minora with our thumb and index finger. Nip the cotton balls with antiseptic solution to disinfect first from the meatus downward and then on the either side, using a new swab for each stroke. Once the meatus is disinfected, do not allow the labia to close over it. The disinfecting order is from inside to outside, and from front to back.	

（续表）

c. Gently insert the catheter into the urinary meatus about 4 - 6 cm, until urine flows. Do not use force to introduce the catheter. If the catheter resists entry, ask the patient to breathe deeply and rotate the catheter slightly. Insert the catheter in the direction of urethra. Then insert the catheter 1 to 2 cm more. d. Place cotton balls and hemostat forceps used into the kidney basin. Move the kidney basin to the edge of the kit. Maintain the nondominant hand in this position throughout the procedure.	—I will sterile your private part, it may be a little cold, take it easy.
（8）Introduce the urine into the treatment bowl. Collect urine specimen. If the treatment bowl is full of urine, nip the catheter and pour the urine into the bedpan. Empty or partially drain the bladder, for adults experiencing urinary retention, some orders limit the amount of urine drained to 1 000 ml.	—Now, please relax and take a deep breath slowly, I will insert the catheter.
（9）Remove the catheter and dry the patient's perineum with gauze. （10）Remove the gloves and assemble equipment. Promote patient comfort. Assist the patient to put on trousers and make patient comfortable. Arrange the top bedcovers and unit in order. （11）Record the time of the catheterization, the amount of urine, the patient's reaction to the procedure, and your name, then label sterile specimen for bacterial culture.	—Now I'm going to remove the catheter. —Thanks for your cooperation. Let me help you with your pants. How about this position? Have a good rest please.

Requirements

1. The nurse can communicate with the patients effectively to make them understand the aims and precautions of inserting the tube Patients cooperation with the nurse actively.

2. The patient is not painful and has no damage to the mucous membrane of urethra.

3. The clothes and lines are not soiled.

4. The nurse has carried out the procedure expertly and correctly and insisted on the sterile principles during the procedure.

5. Finish the procedure in the given time correctly and the patient is satisfied with insertion.

Precautions

1. The equipment should be sterilized strictly and the procedure should be carried out with the aseptic technique.

2. Keep the patient's privacy and explain the procedure to the patient.

3. Select appropriate catheters for patients. Carry out the procedure gently to avoid damaging the mucous membrane of the urethra.

4. Change a new catheter, if inserting a catheter into a female vagina by mistake.

5. For weak adult patients experiencing urinary retention, limit the amount of urine drained to 1 000 ml, which can avoid collapse and hematuria.

Words and Expressions

urinary/ˈjʊərənerɪ/*adj*.尿的;泌尿器的;泌尿的

catheterization/kæθɪraɪˈzeɪʃən/*n*.插管术,导尿术

bladder/ˈblædə/*n*.膀胱

sterile/ˈsterəl/*adj*.无菌的;不毛的,贫瘠的;不生育的;无效果的

perineal/perɪˈnɪrl/*adj*.会阴的

antiseptic/ˌæntɪˈseptɪk/*adj*.防腐的;无菌的;异常洁净的;诚实无欺的;

n.防腐剂,杀菌剂,消毒剂

Critical Thinking

Work in pairs and discuss the following questions.

1. What are the indications for suprapubic catheterization?
2. What factors can influence urination?
3. What are the indications for the use of urinary catheters?
4. How should we prevent the catheter-related problem—UTI(urinary tract infection,尿路感染)?

Unit 7

Obstetric and Gynecological Nursing

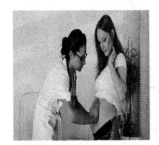 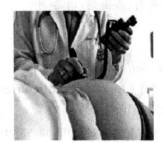 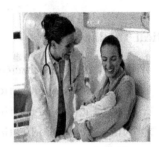

Part I Text

Warming-up

1. What is the goal of the postpartum nursing care?
2. What do the nursing interventions in the postpartum period include?
3. What does the health maintenance in the postpartum period include?

Topic-related Terms

Match the words in Column A with their meanings in Column B.

Column A	Column B
1. postpartum	a. the general region between the anus and the genital organs
2. lochia	b. phlebitis in conjunction with the formation of a blood clot (thrombus)
3. puerperium	c. a natural body passageway
4. thrombophlebitis	d. time period following childbirth when the mother's uterus shrinks and the other functional and anatomic changes of pregnancy are resolved
5. uterus involution	e. substance discharged from the vagina (cellular debris and mucus and blood) that gradually decreases in amount during the weeks following childbirth

（续表）

6. meatus	f. occurring immediately after birth
7. gastrocolic reflex	g. the process by which the uterus and the other genital organs return to their normal pre-pregnant state in the postpartum
8. perineum	h. one of a number of physiological reflexes controlling the motility, or peristalsis, of the gastrointestinal tract

Nursing Care in the Postpartum Period

Nursing care during the postpartum period should consider the physical and psychological needs of mothers and families. The nurse must accurately observe the mother's physiologic functioning and provide timely and focused nursing interventions. The mother's needs for emotional support must be met, anticipatory guidance and health teaching must be given according to the client's readiness to learn, and the developing relationship between parents and newborn must be enhanced and nurtured. The goals of the postpartum nursing care are to assist the new mother and her family to adapt successfully to the transitions after childbirth and the requirements of parenthood.[①]

1. Observing the Uterus Involution

Nurse should assess the height of fundus [②] and characteristics of lochia[③] many times in the first day. After 24 hours, the fundus and lochia can be less assessed. Otherwise, the mother will need basic information about involution including how to assess lochia and how to locate and palpate the fundus. This information allows her to recognize abnormal signs such prolonged lochia and uterine tenderness, which should be reported to the health care provider.

2. Perineal Care

The most common method is to fill a squeeze bottle with warm water and the perineal spray area from the front toward the back. Water alone or with a small amount of cleansing solution added is used. During this procedure water should be avoided to enter the vagina. Teach the mother: thorough hand washing is required before and after changing pads; unused pads should be stored inside their packages; pads should be applied without touching the side that contacts the perineum; the pads should be applied and removed in a front-to-back direction to prevent contamination of the vagina and perineum.

3. Breast Care

Instruct the breastfeeding mother to wash her nipples with clear water and to avoid soaps that remove the natural lubrication secreted by Montgomery's glands. Keeping the nipples dry between feedings helps prevent tissue damage, and wearing a good bra provides necessary support as breast size increases.[④]

4. Health Maintenance

（1）**Nutrition** Shortly after the delivery, the women may express a desire for something to eat or drink. The postpartum diet should provide for balanced nutrition with enough calories to supply the additional requirements for lactation, if the women will be breastfeeding. Mothers usually have good appetites and become hungry between meals, especially if breastfeeding. Between-meal snack, including milk or milk product will help to supply mother with the additional milk requirements to meet mother's needs. An increased intake of fluids is essential for lactating mothers.

(2) **Rest and Sleep**　During the puerperium, the mother needs adequate rest and should be encouraged to relax and sleep whenever possible. Group assessments and care, and try to correlate them with times when the mother would be awake, such as just before or after meals, infant feeding times, and visiting hours. If the room is shared, providing care for both women at the same time also reduces activities that interrupt sleep. A quiet, softly lit environment also promotes sleep.

(3) **Early Ambulation and Exercises**　It is important that the nurse explain the purpose and value of early ambulation to the mother or other decision makers. Activity should be gradually increased according to the mother's strength. Early ambulation promotes circulation and reduces the risk of thrombophlebitis. Bladder and bowel functions will be improved by ambulation, reducing the need for catheterization and decreasing abdomen distention and constipation.

All women should become familiar with exercises after delivery. These movements strengthen the pubococcygeal muscle, which surrounds the vagina and urinary meatus. The exercise involves contracting muscles around the vagina and helps prevent the loss of muscle tone that can occur after childbirth. The exercise is practiced according to mother's health condition gradually. It can be started 2 days after childbirth. One section is practiced in every 1 to 2 days. The frequencies of a section are 8 to 16 times.

(4) **Hygiene**　Taking a shower is refreshing and promotes hygiene. Mothers with no complications are allowed to shower within a few hours of delivery. The first time the mother takes a shower, the nurse should remain nearby for safety. In association with showers, the nurse provides self-care instructions for bathing and breast care.

Emphasize the importance of thoroughly washing her hands before the woman touches her breasts, after diaper changes, after bladder and bowel elimination, and always before handling the infant. This also is emphasized to parents when they see nurses performing careful hand washing.

(5) **Promoting Regular Bowel Elimination**　Adequate fluid and dietary fiber are effective means of preventing constipation. Fruits and vegetables, particularly when they are unpeeled provide dietary fiber act as a natural laxative. Additional fiber is found in whole grain cereals, bread and pasta. Progressive exercise, walking perhaps is the best exercise, and the distance can be increased as strength and endurance increase. Drinking at least 3,000 ml water a day helps maintain normal bowel elimination. A regular schedule of bowel elimination also is important in overcoming constipation. For instance bowel

elimination after breakfast allows the mother to take advantage of the gastrocolic reflex. In addition，measures that reduce perineal and hemorrhoidal pain such as sitz baths and ointments facilitate bowel elimination.

Words and Expressions

postpartum/ˌpəʊstˈpɑːtəm/*adj.*产后的

lochia/ˈləʊkɪə/*n.*恶露(分娩后的子宫阴道分泌物)

puerperium/ˌpjuːəˈpɪərɪəm/*n.*产后期;产褥期

perineal/perɪˈniːəl/*adj.*会阴的

vagina/vəˈdʒaɪnə/*n.*阴道

breastfeeding/brestˈfiːdɪŋ/*v.*用母乳喂养,哺乳

appetite/ˈæpɪtaɪt/*n.*胃口,食欲

thrombophlebitis/ˌθrɒmbəʊflɪˈbaɪtɪs/*n.*血栓(性)静脉炎

catheterization/kæθɪraɪˈzeɪʃən/*n.*插管术,导尿术

constipation/ˌkɒnstɪˈpeɪʃən/*n.*便秘

complications/ˌkɒmplɪˈkeɪʃəns/*n.*并发症

pubococcygeal/pʌbəkɒksɪdˈʒiːl/*adj.*耻骨尾骨的

meatus/mɪˈeɪtəs/*n.*道;口;管

gastrocolic/ˌgæstrəʊˈkɒlɪk/*adj.*连接胃与结肠的

uterus involution 子宫复旧

tissue damage/ˈtɪʃuːˈdæmɪdʒ/组织损伤

abdomen distention 腹胀

gastrocolic reflex 胃肠反射

sitz baths 坐浴

Notes

① 母亲角色转换是指分娩以后,产妇护理新生儿的能力逐步体现,最后能良好地适应母亲角色的过程。母亲角色的转换从妊娠期开始持续到产后几个月,其角色转换包括角色想象阶段、事实角色初始阶段、角色默契阶段和角色实现阶段。

② 子宫底高度因为膀胱充盈会使子宫底升高,在评估子宫底高度时应先让产妇排空膀胱,平躺于床上,评估者一手放在耻骨联合上方,另一只手在脐部轻轻按压子宫直到在腹部扪及一圆、硬的包块即是子宫底,产后1小时内,子宫底平脐或稍升高,以后每天下降1厘米或者1指宽,产后10天,子宫降到盆腔,在耻骨联合上不能扪及。分娩后收缩较好的宫底,应为一硬、圆、光滑的块状物;如宫底软则提示子宫收缩乏力或子宫复旧不良。

③ 大约从产后4天开始,恶露变成粉红色,且量也逐渐减少,这时的恶露称之为浆性恶露;大约产后7~10天后,恶露变成黄色或者白色,称白色恶露。白色恶露大概持续3周,标志子宫内膜已修复正常,正常恶露一般为血腥味,如果在浆性或白色恶露时期出现血性恶露,说明产妇可能有感染或出血,如恶露有味也提示宫腔感染的可能。

④ 乳房产后1~2天,乳房较软,以后乳房的变化主要取决于产妇的哺乳状况。

Text Exploration

Decide whether the following sentence is true or false. If it is true, put "T" in the bracket, if it is false, put "F" in the bracket.

1. The goals of the postpartum nursing care are to assist the new mother and her family to adapt successfully to the transitions after childbirth and the requirements of parenthood. (   )
2. The most common method for perineal care is to fill a squeeze bottle with warm water and the perineal spray area from the front toward the back. (   )
3. The mother should not wear a good bra provides necessary support as breast size increases. (   )
4. During the puerperium, the mother needs adequate rest and should be encouraged to relax and sleep whenever possible. (   )
5. All women should not become familiar with exercises after delivery. (   )

Part Ⅱ Dialogue ....

Read the following dialogue. Then do Role-play task by using the Sentence Models with your partner.

(Zhang Ling and her instructress Ms. Jiang are examining Mrs. Li, a primipara, who has labor pains. An hour later.)

Ms. Jiang: Mrs. Li, I think it's time to go to the delivery room. Zhang Ling, please help her.

Zhang Ling: OK. Mrs. Li, you can lean on me. Don't worry.

Mrs. Li: Thank you. I feel so weak and dizzy.

Zhang Ling: That's normal. Just sit down on the bed here.

Ms. Jiang: Mrs. Li is there a cramp coming? Let's wait until it passes. Open your mouth quickly and shallowly. Did the pain go away?

Mrs. Li: I think so.

Ms. Jiang: Then you can lie down. Move your buttocks towards the end, and put your feet in the stirrups. When the next cramp comes, you can start pushing down. Wait until you can't hold it any longer and then start pushing down, just like when you go to the toilet.

Mrs. Li: There's another cramp coming.

Ms. Jiang: Take a deep breath and push! Push harder! Take another breath and push again! Once more! Is the pain gone?

Mrs. Li: Yes.

Ms. Jiang: Then let's wait for the next one.

Mrs. Li: Oh, here it comes again.

Ms. Jiang: Take a deep breath and push down! Hard! Just a bit more! Well done!

Zhang Ling: Oh, I see the baby's head.

(The second morning after the delivery.)

Ms. Jiang: Congratulations, Mrs. Li! Here is the baby boy. Did you sleep well?

Mrs. Li: Yes, very well, thank you.

Ms. Jiang: I'd like to check the fundus of your uterus to see how well it is contracted. Is there much blood?

Mrs. Li: Just a bit.

Ms. Jiang: Could I have a look at your sanitary pad to see the lochia? Do you know how to clean your perineal area?

Mrs. Li: No.

Ms. Jiang: Zhang Ling, come on, please help Mrs. Li clean the perineal area.

Zhang Ling: OK. Use a clean, wet cloth and wipe towards your anus. So from the front to the back, never the opposite way.

Mr. Chen: Yes, I see.

Ms. Jiang: How's the breast-feeding going?

Mrs. Li: The baby's sucking well but I don't have much milk.

Ms. Jiang: That will come soon. Make sure that you put the baby's tongue well under your nipple, and then you use one hand to keep the breast in his mouth. You may feel some cramps in your uterus when you are feeding him, but that's very normal. Whenever you have some questions, please ask me anytime.

Mrs. Li: Thank you very much.

Words and Expressions

primipara/praɪˈmɪpərə/ *n.* 初产的孕妇

delivery/dɪˈlɪvərɪ/ *n.* 分娩

dizzy/ˈdɪzɪ/ *adj.* 晕眩的；使人头晕的

stirrup/ˈstɪrəp/ *n.* 足蹬

cramp/kræmp/ *n.* 痉挛，腹痛

fundus/ˈfʌndəs/ *n.* 基底；底部

uterus/ˈjuːtərəs/ *n.* 子宫

push down 下推；向下推

Sentence Models

Take a deep breath and push!

Did you sleep well?

I'd like to check the fundus of your uterus to see how well it is contracted.

Could I have a look at your sanitary pad to see the lochia?

How's the breast-feeding going?

Make sure that you put the baby's tongue well under your nipple, and then you use one hand to keep the breast in his mouth.

Role-play

Make a dialogue. Student A acts as a primipara who hasn't much milk and doesn't know how to feed her baby; student B acts as a nurse who is going to tell her what to do. Use the above Sentence Models as guidelines.

Part III Scene Practice

Read the information below about Aseptic technique. Make sure about the correct ways and procedures. Student A acts as a patient; Student B acts as a nurse and then practise this action with the equipment prepared. Do use the expressions to communicate with each other effectively.

Performing Practices of Asepsis

Aseptic technique is used to prevent microorganisms from invading human beings, sterile articles and sterile fields from being contaminated during medical procedures and nursing interventions. Aseptic techniques are used to reduce the risk of post-procedure infections and to minimize the exposure of health care providers to potentially infectious microorganisms.

Purposes

1. To maintain sterile articles and sterile area sterile.

2. To halt the spread of microorganisms and minimize the threat and disease of infection.

Preparing

1. **Nurse** Wear the uniform round cap, shoes and mask. Fail nails short and wash hands before aseptic procedures, wear sterile gloves if it is necessary.

2. **Equipment** Sterile container and sterile forceps, dressing jar, swabs, disinfectant, sterile solution, sterile package, a sterile bowl, square plate containing sterile articles, sterile gloves, emesis basin, bottle opener, pen and paper cleaning cloth, two clean trays. Assemble equipment and arrange on a nursing cart in the order of their use.

3. **Environment** The environment should be clean, dry and bright. The field where the aseptic technique is operated should be clean, roomy and dry. Stop sweeping to keep indoor air fresh. Avoid raising dust, which may carry organisms.

Standards and Procedure

Action

1. Gather equipment. Check that sterile wrapped drape or package is dry and unopened. Also note expiration date.

2. Select a work area that is waist level or higher. Open sterile wrapped drape by folding the topmost part of the covering wrapper away from you. Next, open the sides of the set. Remove forceps from the container, keep the prongs together and lift the forceps without touching any part of the container. The forceps' tips need to be held down, particularly if they become wet, so that fluid will not flow from a contaminated area to a sterile one. As with other sterile objects, forceps should be kept above waist level. Remove a sterile drape from the sterile package. Gently tap the prongs together directly over the container to remove excess solution. Fold the sterile package as it is.

3. Apply the sterile treatment tray with one drape.

(1) Hold the outer surface of the one side of the drape at about 2 cm from the edge of unilateral drape with one hand, hold the other side of the drape at the same area with the other hand, gently open and place the drape with double folds in the tray; hold the outer surface of the upper layer of the drape at two corners with both hands and fanfold it with its edge toward outside.

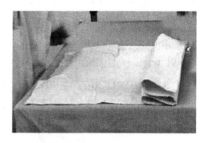

(2) Place additional sterile items on field as needed. Fold the opening end of drape twice upward, tuck the sides of the drape in and record the date and time of applying the tray. The aseptic tray is considered as sterile for 4 hours.

(3) Wrap the sterile package with one tape and write the opening date and time in the label or paper of the package when the sterile items are still left. The sterile package opened and uncontaminated is considered as sterile for 24 hours.

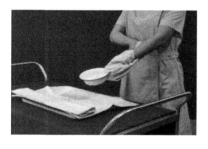

4. Apply the sterile treatment tray with two drapes.

(1) Read the label on the sterile package and open the sterile package as the same way as applying the sterile treatment tray with one drape. Hold the outside of the drape at two corners with both hands, gently open and place it in the tray evenly from opposite side of the tray to near side and make the sterile side upward.

(2) Pick up the sterile bowl package with the left hand, open the sterile bowel and drop it onto the sterile field from a safe distance, being careful that the outside wrapper does not touch the sterile field. The nondominant hand should be used to secure the loose ends away from the item and protect them from contaminating the sterile field.

(3) Check the sterile solution carefully. Remove the cap carefully. Pour a small amount of the solution into waste container to clean the lip of the bottle. Be sure the label side of the container is uppermost when pouring so that the label does not become wet and soiled. Pour carefully so as not to splash the solution. Touch only the outside of the cap when recapping.

(4) Place additional sterile items on field as needed.

（5）Remove a sterile drape with a sterile forceps. Hold the outside of the drape at two corners with both hands, gently open and place it in the tray evenly from near to off side and fold them upward.

（6）Once a solution has been opened, the outer bottle should be labeled and dated if it is to be reused. Most solutions are considered sterile for 24 hours after they are opened.

（7）Place sterile glove package on clean, dry surface above your waist. Expose the sterile gauze by open a part of the drape. Carefully open the inner package and expose the sterile gloves with the cuff closed to you. Grasp edge of folded cuff. Lift and hold gloves with fingers down. Pull first glove on with cuff folded. Slide fingers of gloved hand under cuff of second glove. Insert hand with cuff folded. Adjust gloves on both hands. Lift up the gauze from the tray, wipe the talcum powder on the gloves and then hold the sterile bowl with both hands.

（8）Invert glove as it is removed. Slide ungloved fingers inside second glove. Remove second glove inside out. Discard gloves in appropriate container and wash hands.

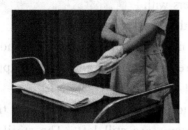 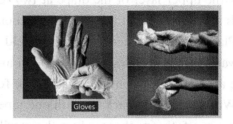

5. Dispose of the equipment used.

Words and Expressions

aseptic/eɪˈseptɪk/ *adj*. 无菌的；防感染的
microorganism/maɪkrəʊˈɔːg(ə)nɪz(ə)m/ *n*. 微生物
mask/mɑːsk/ *n*. 面具；口罩
forceps/ˈfɔːseps; -sɪps/ *n*. 钳子
sterile container 无菌容器
sterile package 无菌包
grasp/ɡrɑːsp/ *vt*. 抓住；领会
dispose/dɪˈspəʊz/ *vt*. 处理

Critical Thinking

Work in pairs and discuss the following questions.

1. Why are aseptic techniques important?
2. What are principles of aseptic technique?
3. What are the methods of aseptic technique?
4. What should be noted for using sterile package?

Unit 8

Pediatric Nursing

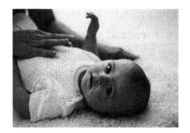 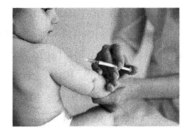 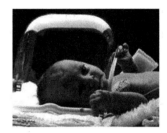

Part I Text ....

Warming-up

1. What are the relief measures applied in reducing elevated temperature?
2. Could you tell us the process of physical cooling approach?

Topic-related Terms

Match the words in Column A their definitions in with Column B.

Column A	Column B
1. pediatric	a. of or relating to the medical care of children
2. defervescence	b. depletion of bodily fluids
3. pyrogen	c. the part of the face above the eyes
4. dehydration	d. abatement of a fever
5. forehead	e. any substance that can cause a rise in body temperature
6. antipyretic	f. noun: any medicine that lowers body temperature to prevent or alleviate fever adjective: preventing or alleviating fever
7. influenza	g. purchasable without a doctor's prescription
8. nonprescription	h. an acute febrile highly contagious viral disease

Pediatric Nursing—Reducing Elevated Temperature

The principal reason for treating fever is the relief of discomfort; no specific degree of fever requires treatment. Nurse should first notify physician of fever, administer antipyretic drugs as ordered. Monitor infant's fluid intake and urine output to prevent dehydration. Relief measures include pharmacologic and/or physical intervention.

The process of physical cooling approach is: (a) expose the skin to the air. If the environment is warm, a fan or an air conditioner may be turned on but the draft should not be directly on the child; (b) ice bags can be placed in the forehead and axillas, wrap the ice bag with clothes or use 30% - 50% alcohol to stroke the forehead and extremity; (c) administer a tepid bath: prepare a basin of tepid water (32 - 34°C) with towels and washcloth. Monitor vital signs before staring. Place cool, moist cloths under each axilla, groin and on forehead. Bath each extremity using long strokes. Use friction gently, to bring the blood to the surface. Change water as necessary to keep water tepid; (d) continue this procedure until temperature is reduced; (e) take vital signs 30 minutes after the end of the sponge bath.

Antipyretic drugs include acetaminophen, aspirin, and nonsteroidal anti-inflammatory drugs (NSAIDs). Acetaminophen is the preferred drug; aspirin should not be given to children because of the possible association between aspirin use in children with influenza virus or chickenpox and Reye syndrome. Dosage is based on the initial temperature level: 5mg/kg of body weight for temperatures less than 39.2°C (102.5 °F) or 10mg/kg for temperatures greater than 39.2°C (102.5 °F). The recommended dosage for pain is 10mg/kg every 6 to 8 hours, and the recommended maximum daily does for pain and fever is 40mg/kg. The duration of fever reduction is generally 6 to 8 hours. Nonprescription ibuprofen (Advil, Nuprin, Motrin IB, Medipren) is not approved for use in children under 12 years of age.

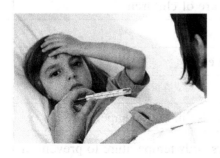

It should be given every 4 hours, but no more than five times in 24 hours. Since body temperature normally decreases at night, three to four doses in 24 hours will usually control most fevers. The temperature is usually retaken 30 minutes after the antipyretic is given to assess its effect but should not be repeatedly measured. The child's level of discomfort is the best indication for continued treatment.

Seizures associated with a fever occur in 3% to 4% of all children, usually in those between 3 months and 5 years of age. For children who have febrile seizures, administration of antipyretics does not prevent recurrences.

Words and Expressions

fever/ˈfiːvə/ n . 发烧,发热

antipyretic/ˌæntɪpaɪˈretɪk/ n . (药)退热剂

forehead/ˈfɔːhed/ n . 额,前额

axillas/ækˈsɪləz/ n . [解剖]腋窝,[解剖]腋下;胳肢窝

seizures/ˈsiːʒəs/ n . 癫痫,痉挛;发作(seizure 的复数)

nonprescription/ˌnɒnprɪˈskrɪpʃən/ adj . 非处方的;未经医生处方可以买到的

chickenpox/ˈtʃɪkɪnpɑks/ n . 〈内科〉水痘

Notes

① 被动语态由"助动词 be＋及物动词的过去分词"构成。例如：It should be given every 4 hours...

② 退热剂用量以最初的体温水平为基础：低于 39.2℃(102.5℉),每千克体重 5 毫克;高于 39.2℃,每千克体重 10 毫克。

③ 患儿应用阿司匹林可能与感染流行性感冒病毒或水痘及 Reye 综合征有关,因此阿司匹林不应该给患儿应用。

④ 降温的方法包括药物降温和物理降温。

⑤ febrile seizure   高热惊厥

Text Exploration

Decide whether the following sentence is true or false . If it is true，put "T" in the bracket，if it is false，put "F" in the bracket .

1. One of physical cooling approaches is ice bags can be placed in the forehead and axillas, wrap the ice bag with clothes. (   )

2. Antipyretic drugs include aspirin, acetaminophen, and nonsteroidal anti-inflammatory drugs. (   )

3. Aspirin should be given to children because of the possible association between aspirin use in children with influenza virus or chickenpox and Reye syndrome. (   )

4. Antipyretic drugs should be given every 4 hours，but no more than six times in 24 hours. (   )

5. The temperature is usually retaken 30 minutes after the antipyretic is given to assess its effect but should not be repeatedly measured. (   )

Part Ⅱ   Dialogue ···

Read the following dialogue . Then do the Role-Play task by using the sentence Models with your partner .

Care for the Child with Pneumonia

Nurse: Mrs. Brown, is your baby getting any better?

Child's Parent: No, she seems to be getting worse.

Nurse: Is her coughing better?

Child's Parent: Yes.

Nurse: Some baby patients have dry paroxysmal cough at the early stage of pneumonia. As time goes on, the disintegrated granulocytes and dead bacteria and virus become sputum, which will stimulate the bronchi and result in paroxysmal cough and sputum. It is like a battle field where lays many dead enemy soldiers. Sputum is the waste product that is being cleaned from the body's respiratory system. There is a disease development process.

Child's Parent: She has had the intravenous transfusion for 3-4 days without any improvement.

Nurse: You should not worry too much. We are giving the baby a very effective treatment, but it takes time for the drugs to take effects. Let's try to be a little more patient, OK?

Child's Parent: We are very worried for our only baby since she has been ill for more than 7 days.

Nurse: I can understand how you feel. However, your worries cannot solve any problems. Rather, it will affect your own immune system. You should take better care of yourself.

Child's Parent: Then what should I pay attention to?

Nurse: At home you should often open the windows and keep the air fresh. When your baby coughs, pat her back softly to help her cough up the sputum. When patting, you should close your five fingers of your hand and pat on the baby's back with only the edge of the hand. Pat her softly and let the vibration from the patting to help the baby cough up her sputum (Demonstrated how to pat).

Child's Parent: OK, I get it.

Nurse: Since your baby is too young to spit, she can only swallow it. When you find some mucus in her stool, it's the sputum she had swallowed.

Child's Parent: Oh, now I see. I thought it was the bad food she ate.

Nurse: Sometimes because the sputum stimulates the gastrointestinal track or due to the virus's effect, some babies will have diarrhea. But you need not worry too much because not every baby has diarrhea. Since your baby has a fever, we'll take her temperature every 4 hours. Please call us to measure her temperature at any time if you feel she has a fever. If her temperature is too high, the doctor will give her an antipyretic drug. Please don't give her any medicine yourself. Feed your baby more water and change her clothes when she is perspiring too much. You may put a dry towel on her back to prevent her from catching cold. I will come around some time later. You may press the call button to call us if you need us.

Words and Expressions

pneumonia/njuːˈməʊnɪə/ n. 肺炎

paroxysmal/ˌpærəkˈsɪzməl/ adj. 发作性的,爆发性的;阵发性的

dry paroxysmal cough 阵发性干咳

granulocytes/ˈɡrænjʊləsaɪts/ n. 〈医〉粒性白细胞

bacteria/bækˈtɪərɪə/ n. 细菌(bacterium 的名词复数)

sputum/ˈspjuːtəm/ n. 痰(复数:sputa)

bronchi/ˈbrɒŋkaɪ/ n. 支气管;(尤指肺两侧的)支气管(bronchus 的名词复数)

Sentence Models

Is your baby getting better?

Is her coughing better?

We are giving the baby a very effective treatment,but it takes time for the drugs to take effects.

Let's try to be a little more patient,OK?

When your baby coughs,pat her back softly to help her cough up the sputum.

When patting,you should close your five fingers of your hand and pat on the baby's back with only the edge of the hand.

Since your baby has a fever,we'll take her temperature every 4 hours.

Please call us to measure her temperature at any time if you feel she has a fever.

I will come around some time later.

You may press the call button to call us if you need us.

Role-play

Make a dialogue. Student A acts as a parent of a sick child; student B acts as a nurse who is going to talk about the child's condition with student A.

Use the useful sentence patterns as guidelines.

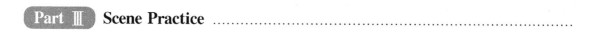

Part Ⅲ Scene Practice

Administering Oxygen

Administering Oxygen by an Oxygen Cylinder

Purposes

1. To decrease shortness of breath and fatigue (tiredness).

2. To improve sleep in some people who have sleep-related breathing disorders.

3. To improve the lifespan of some people who have COPD.

Preparing

1. Nurse: Wear the uniform, nurse's cap and shoes. Wash your hands.

2. Patient: Make the patient understand the aims of administering oxygen and cooperate with the nurse actively.

3. Equipment: A treatment tray with a cup of cold boiled water, sterile gauze, a wrench, emesis basin, sterile nasal catheters, glass connector, sterile swabs, adhesive tapes, safety pin, alcohol or turpentine, record sheet, pen, oxygen cylinder and oxygen gauge tubing. Assemble equipment and arrange on the nursing cart in the order of their use.

4. Environment: Keep away from any source of fire and heat. No smoking in the ward. Forbid placing the pyrotechnical and tinderbox near the oxygen cylinder. Move the stove from the oxygen cylinder about 5 metres, and from a radiator about 1 metre.

Standards and Procedures

Action	Nursing Expression
1. Install oxygen gauge 　1) Check the "full" sign and remove the safety cap. 　2) With the outlet pointing away from you and others, open the cylinder valve slightly and close it quickly. This blows away dust from the valve opening. 　3) Insert the regulator inlet into the valve opening and tighten the nut with a wrench. 　4) Attach the humidifier, rubbing and glass connector to the flowmeter. 　5) Turn the regulator adjustment knob fully to the off position. This must be done before turning the cylinder valve on. 　6) Open the cylinder valve slowly. Check that oxygen is flowing out of glass connector. 2. Assemble equipment and explain procedure to patient and family. 3. Examine the patient's nostrils and clear them with soaked water swab. Prepare the adhesive tapes. 4. Attach the catheter to the oxygen supply and to the humidifier. Start the oxygen at the prescribed rate. Note that oxygen is being delivered properly by placing the end of the catheter in a glass of water. 5. Measure the 2/3 distance from the nostril to the earlobe as a guide for the distance to insert the catheter. Insert the catheter by moving it carefully along the floor of the nose until the measured distance is reached. Secure it to the patient with adhesive. The tubing from the oxygen supply may be secured to the bed linen with a pin.	—Hello, Mrs. Li. I'd like to supply oxygen to decrease shortness of your breath. OK? —Let me clean your nostrils. —Now, I'll insert the nasal catheter for you.

（续表）

6. Check the flow of oxygen regularly and maintain it at the prescribed rate. Finish the record sheet. Explain precaution to the patient.	—Now, we're through. You know, oxygen is a kind of flammable and combustible gas. And remember that: No smoking here. Don't adjust the flow rate by yourself, it's a dangerous thing. OK? I'll check on you often. Thanks, Mrs. Brown. Um, just ring when you want me to observe you.
7. Observe patient's response to therapy. 8. Stop applying oxygen 　1）Identify patient and explain the reason of stopping providing oxygen to the patient. 　2）Remove the catheter with gauze. 　3）Turn off the cylinder valve and remove oxygen completely. 　4）Remove the catheter. 　5）Turn the regulator adjustment knob fully to the off position. 9. Assist patient to a comfortable position. 10. Record the time of stopping applying oxygen and signature. 11. Dispose of the equipment used.	—Hello, Mrs. Brown. How are you? Now, your condition is well in hand. The lips are not blue, the face is rosy, and the breath is steady. I'll remove oxygen for you, okay? —Now, you need a rest. Bye!

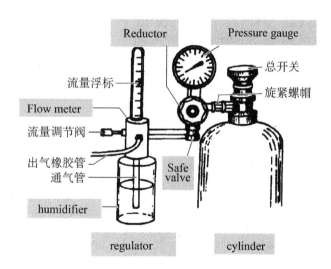

Administering Oxygen by Wall Oxygen Setup

Purpose

1. To decrease shortness of breath and fairing (tiredness).

2. To improve sleep in some people who have sleep-related breathing disorders.

3. To improve the lifespan of some people who have COPD.

Preparing

1. Nurse: Wear the uniform, nurse's cap and shoes. Wash your hands.

2. Patient: Explain the aims to the patient. Let the patient understand the notes of the procedure and make ready for it.

3. Equipment: Sterile gauze, oxygen gauge, nasal cannula, a cup of cold boiled water, emesis basin, sterile swabs, record sheet, pen. Assemble equipment and arrange on the nursing cart in the order of their use.

4. Environment: Keep away from any source of fire and heat. No smoking in the ward. Forbid placing the pyrotechnical and tinderbox near the oxygen cylinder. Move the stove from the oxygen cylinder about 5 metres, and from a radiator about 1 metre.

Standards and Procedure

Action	Nursing Expression
1. Assemble equipment and explain procedure to patient and family.	—Hello, Lily. I'd like to supply oxygen to decrease shortness your of breath. OK?
2. Examine the patient's nostrils and clear them with soaked water swab.	—Let me clean your nostrils.
3. Plug the flowmeter into the wall outlet and attach the humidifier to the flowmeter. Connect the nasal cannula to the oxygen setup.	
4. Adjust the flow rate as ordered by physician. Check that oxygen is flowing out of prongs by placing the end of the catheter in a glass of water.	
5. Place the prongs in the nostrils. Over and behind each ear with adjuster comfortably under chin or around the patient's head.	—I'll place it in your nostrils.
6. Finish the record sheet. Instruct the patient to breathe through his nose.	
7. Explain precautions to the patient.	—Now, we're through. You know, Oxygen is a kind of flammable and combustible gas. And remember that: No smoking here. Don't adjust the flow rate by yourself, it's a dangerous thing. OK? I'll check on you often. Thanks, Lily. Um, just ring when you want me to observe you.
8. Observe patient's response to therapy.	
9. Stop applying oxygen.	
1) Identify patient and explain the reason of stopping providing oxygen to the patient.	
2) Remove the cannula. Turn it off.	
3) Record the time of stopping applying oxygen and signature.	—Hello, Lily. How are you? Now, your condition is well in hand. The lips are not blue, the face is rosy, and the breath is steady. Then I'll remove oxygen for you, OK?
10. Dispose of the equipment used and assist patient to a comfortable position.	—Now, you need a good rest. Bye!

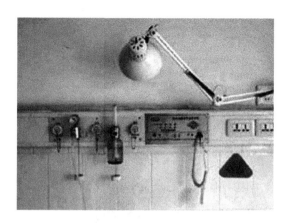

Words and Expressions

Oxygen Cylinder　氧气瓶	Safe Valve　安全阀
Oxygen Regulator　氧气表	Nasal Catheter　鼻腔导管
Pressure Gauge　压力表	Nasal Cannula　鼻塞
Redactor　减压器	Oxygen Mask　氧气面罩
Flowmeter　流量表	Wall Oxygen Setup/Wall Outlet Supply
Humidifier　湿化瓶	中心供氧装置

Critical Thinking

Work in pairs and discuss the following questions.

1. What's the purpose of administering Oxygen?
2. How should you do to ensure the safe use of administering Oxygen by an Oxygen Cylinder?
3. What should you pay attention to when administering Oxygen by an Oxygen Cylinder?
4. How do you judge that hypoxia has improved?

Unit 9

Discharge

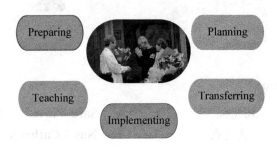

Part Ⅰ **Text** ....

Warming-up

1. Are you eager to go home if you have been in hospital for some time due to certain disease?
2. What does a patient in hospital do when he pulls through his illness?
3. What should a nurse do for a patient to be charged from hospital?

Topic-related Terms

Please match the words in Column A with their definitions in Column B.

Column A	Column B
1. discharge	a. being careful to avoid danger or mistakes
2. schedule	b. meeting with a doctor to get his advice
3. caution	c. give official permission for (somebody) to leave
4. instruction	d. reduce something to the smallest possible amount or degree
5. ensure	e. arrange something for a certain time
6. minimize	f. make it certain that something will happen
7. coordinate	g. a statement telling someone what they must do
8. consultation	h. organize an activity so that the people involved in it work well and achieve a good result

Discharge

When a patient is discharged from hospital, he is officially allowed to leave after going through necessary procedures.[①] Generally speaking, discharge is the last program for an in-patient in hospitals. It is necessary for a nurse to make a discharge plan and do discharge teaching for a patient who is about to be discharged.

Discharge Planning

Discharge planning is a routine feature of health systems in many countries. It is the development of an individualized discharge plan for the patient prior to leaving the hospital.[②] It may ensure that patients are discharged at an appropriate time and provided with adequate post-discharge services. It is a process that aims to improve the coordination of services after discharge from hospital by considering the patient's needs in the community. It seeks to bridge the gap between hospital and the place to which the patient is discharged, reduce length of stay in hospital, and minimize unplanned readmission to hospital[③]. Discharge planning involves close collaboration between the patient, the family, and the multidisciplinary team[④] helping the patient to get assistance with the care they will need when they leave the acute hospital. The nurses should plan ahead for the patient's discharge by doing the following:

1. Including the patient and family as full partners in the discharge planning process.
2. Letting the patient and family understand his health and having timely and accurate communication for discharge.
3. Planning the date and time of discharge early.
4. Planning for patients to be discharged before the peak in admissions.
5. Coordinating and checking everything is in place 48 hours before discharge to ensure that everything is ready.

Discharge Teaching

A patient is rarely completely well at the time he leaves the hospital, and he must still have a period of recovery. For the patient to fully recover, a nurse, who is responsible for offering the necessary instructions to a patient and his family, must manage to make him understand and remember the following instructions (list and print them for the patient) as soon as she knows the patient is about to be discharged.

1. Next consultation. Tell the patient the day, the date and time for the next scheduled visit to the clinic for a consultation. Remind him to get advice from the doctor when he needs it.
2. The medication. Inform how and when to take medication. Explain the need for care, caution and accuracy. Teach him to do it exactly as you say.
3. The diet. Describe the diet as simply as possible. Name the foods that are not allowed, the foods that are necessary every day, and the amounts allowed.
4. Reduction of risk factors. Tell him that taking medication is only one part of his

treatment regime，and that reducing other risk factors is also important：losing weight（if overweight），stopping smoking，avoiding stressful and emotional pressure，etc.

5. Danger signs to watch out for. These may include an abdominal reaction to insulin or other medication；bleeding on the dressings；or prolonged bed rest.

6. Instructions for a bedridden patient. Give instructions to the family about giving a bath，moving and turning the patient，giving the bedpan，etc.

7. Rest and activity. The amount of rest that the patient must have and that the amount of activity he is allowed.

8. They are valuable for the patient's future care after he is discharged.

9. Once the patient has left, the nurse should clean the ward and make an empty bed to receive a new patient.

Words and Expressions

discharge/dɪsˈtʃɑrdʒ/ v.& n. 排出，让走掉，(让)出院

individualize/ˌɪndəˈvɪdʒʊəˌlaɪz/ v. 赋予个性，个性化

coordination/kəʊˌɔːdnˈeɪʃən/ n. 协调，和谐

minimize/ˈmɪnəˌmaɪz/ vt. 把……减至最低数量[程度]，对(某事物)作最低估计

readmission/ˌriːədˈmɪʃən/ n. 重新接纳，重新入场(入院或入学)许可

collaboration/kəˌlæbəˈreɪʃən/ n. 合作，协作，通敌，勾结

multidisciplinary/ˌmʌltɪˈdɪsəpləˌneri/ adj. 包括各种学科的，有关各种学问的，多学科

consultation/ˌkɒnslˈteɪʃən/ n. 咨询；磋商；[临床]会诊；讨论会

schedule/ˈʃedjuːəl//ˈskedʒʊl, -ʊəl/ v.& n. 安排，将……列表，时刻表

instruction/ɪnˈstrʌkʃən/ n. 授，教导；教诲

caution/ˈkɔːʃən/ v.& n. 小心，谨慎，劝告

accuracy/ˈækjʊrəsɪ/ n. 精确(性)，准确(性)

regime/reɪˈʒiːm/ n. 政权，养生法，(病人等的)生活规则

insulin/ˈɪnsəlɪn/ n. 胰岛素

Notes

① (住院)病人在办理了必要的手续之后正式获准离开医院，即出院。

② 它(出院计划)是(医院)在病人出院前为其制定的个性化出院计划。

　　prior to：在……之前

③ 寻求缩小医院和病人出院后落脚处的距离，减少病人住院时间，最大限度地降低病人再入院的几率。

　　to which the patient is discharged 是定语从句，修饰其前面的先行词 the place.

④ 定出院计划需要病人、病人家属和医疗团队密切协作。

Text Exploration

Decide whether the following sentence is true or false. If it is true, put "T" in the bracket, if it is false, put "F" in the bracket.

1. When a patient is about to be discharged, a nurse needn't do anything for him(or her).
    (   )
2. The nurses should plan ahead for the patient's discharge by planning for patients to be discharged before the rush hour in admissions. (   )
3. A patient is usually completely well at the time he leaves the hospital. (   )
4. Discharge instructions are useful for the patient's future care after he is discharged.
    (   )
5. As soon as the patient has been discharged, the nurse should clean the ward and make an empty bed to receive a new patient. (   )

Part Ⅱ **Dialogue** ....

Read the following dialogue. Then do Role-play task by using the Sentence Models with your partner.

Discharge Teaching

(In a ward, Li Mei's instructor, Miss Xie, is demonstrating how to do discharge teaching.)

Nurse: Good morning, Mrs. Zhao. How are you feeling today?

Patient: Good morning, Miss Xie. Splendid.

Nurse: Good. You can be discharged tomorrow. How does it sound?

Patient: Terrific, I'm so eager to go home.

Nurse: Mrs. Zhao, you will need to continue being on a low-salt diet after your discharge.

Patient: Why do I need to continue doing that?

Nurse: You still have high blood pressure. Too much salt can make it worse. So you need to be careful about having salt or sodium.

Patient: I don't add salt to my food now.

Nurse: Good. Many foods have salt in them. Here is a list of foods you should not eat.

Patient: I didn't know that garlic has salt in it.

Nurse: Yes. You need to look at the label. Here is an explanation of your new medicine. It is a diuretic that means it will make you urinate more. This will help your blood pressure under control. The medicine can make you lose potassium, so you need to eat foods that have it.

Patient: Like bananas and oranges?

Nurse: Yes. There is a list of foods that have potassium. Additionally, see this paper which explains you medicine. Notice the first point. If you forget one dose, don't take two doses together. Drink enough fluids. If you have any of the symptoms on this list, call your doctor.

Patient: If I forget a pill, what should I do?

Nurse: You'd better not take two doses together. If you forget your 7:30 a.m. dose, but remember it at 2:30 p.m., don't take your morning dose. Just wait until the usual time and take your afternoon dose then. What time is your afternoon dose?

Patient: At 4:30 p.m. So I would take just one dose that day.

Nurse: Right. Please read over these papers. If you have any question, please ask.

Words and Expressions

demonstrate/ˈdemənstreɪt/ n. 展示；演示，说明

sodium/ˈsəʊdɪəm/ n. 钠（含量）

garlic/ˈgɑːlɪk/ n. (英)大蒜；蒜头

diuretic/ˌdaɪjʊˈretɪk/ n. 利尿剂

urinate/ˈjʊərɪneɪt/ vi. 排尿，撒尿

potassium/pəˈtæsɪəm/ n. (英)钾

dose/dəʊs/ n. 一服，一剂

symptom/ˈsɪmptəm/ n. 症状；征兆

Sentence Models

How are you feeling today?

Splendid. How does it sound?

Terrific, I'm so eager to go home.

If I forget a pill, what should I do? Look at the label.

If you have any question, please ask.

Congratulations. Here is a discharge form for you. Keep a diet of vegetables and fruits.

Take one tablet of this medicine three times a day before meals.

Here is a list of foods you should not eat.

You'd better not take two doses together.

Role-play

Make a dialogue. Student A acts as a patient who needs to be on a fat-free diet resulting from overweight. Student B acts as a senior nurse like Ms. Xie in the dialogue. And student B explains to student A about the fat-free diet. Use the above Sentence Models as guidelines.

Part Ⅲ Scene Practice

Read the information below about transferring a patient from a wheelchair to a car. Make sure about the correct ways and procedures. Student A acts as a patient; students B and C act as nurses and then practice this action with the equipment prepared. Do use the expressions to communicate with each other effectively.

Transferring a Patient from a Wheelchair to a Car

Purpose: to transfer a patient from a wheelchair to a car who can't move on his/her own when being discharged.

Preparing

1. Nurses: Wear the uniform, shoes, nurse's cap and mask. Wash your hands. Explain the procedure to the patient. Make him/her understand the notes of the procedure and make ready for it.

2. Patient: Know something about the action of a wheelchair, understand the notes of the procedure and actively cooperate.

3. Equipment: A wheelchair, paper and a pen.

4. Environment: No obstacles.

Standards and Procedure

Action

1. Open the door of the car.

2. Roll the wheelchair to the car doorway.

3. Adjust the height of the wheelchair.

4. Slowly roll the wheelchair backwards to insert the patient, through the car doorway (being careful to protect his/her head, as it passes through the door frame).

5. Lift the patient from the wheelchair(While one nurse is supporting the patient, the other nurse detaches the strap fasteners(带状扣件)from the wheelchair and slides wheelchair out of the way).

6. Lower the patient onto the car seat.

7. Swing the patient's legs into the car, until the patient is rotated and facing forwards.

8. Close the door of the car.

9. The wheelchair may be folded and put in the car if possible.

Words and Expressions

transfer/trænsˈfɜː/ v. & n. 转移；（旅行中）转乘，转搭；转让

detach/dəˈtætʃ/ v. 拆卸，取下，使分开后将其拿下

fasteners/ˈfɑːstnəz/ n. 扣件

swing/swɪŋ/ v. 摆动；摇动；（借下面支点）纵身一跳；滑动

rotate/rəʊˈteɪt/ vi. 旋转；循环

　　　　　　　vt. 使旋转；使转动；使轮流

Critical Thinking

Work in pairs and discuss the following questions.

1. What is the special requirement for the nurses doing the transferring job?
2. What should be done for a patient's safety before moving him/her?
3. How do you do to make the patient cooperative?
4. Suppose that you are asked to transfer a patient from a bed to a wheelchair，are you sure you can do the job well? How?

METS(二级)样卷(A)

医护英语水平考试

（二级）

Medical English Test System（METS）

Level 2

姓名_____   准考证号_____   时间：120 分钟

考生注意事项

1. 严格遵守考场规则,考生得到监考人员的指令后方可开始答题。

2. 考生须将自己的姓名和准考证号写在本试卷上。

3. 作答前,考生务必将自己的姓名、准考证号用黑色字迹的签字笔填写在答题卡指定位置,并将准考证号对应的信息点用 2B 铅笔涂黑。

4. 全部试题均在答题卡上作答,在试卷上作答无效。选择题部分,用 2B 铅笔把答题卡上对应题目的答案标号涂黑。如需改动,用橡皮擦干净后,再涂选其他答案。非选择题部分,用黑色字迹的签字笔在答题卡的指定位置答题。

5. 考试结束后考生将试题和答题卡放在桌上,不得带走,待监考人员收毕清点后,方可离场。任何个人或机构不得保留、复制和出版本试卷,不得以任何形式传播试卷内容。违者必究。

教育部考试中心

××××年××月

Ⅰ. Listening

Part 1

Questions 1 – 5

You will hear five patients describing their pain to the nurse.

What pain does each patient have?

For questions 1 – 5, mark the correct letter A-H on your answer sheet.

You will hear each conversation twice.

Example:

0. Heath

0	A	B	C	D	E	F	G	H
	□	□	□	□	□	■	□	□

1. Hales	**A.** Sore eye
2. Lan	**B.** Stomachache
3. Jack	**C.** Pain in the leg
4. Swift	**D.** Backache
5. Bloomfield	**E.** Pain in the chest
	F. Pain in the hands
	G. Pain in the forehead
	H. Sore throat

Part 2

Questions 6 – 10

You will hear a conversation between Miles, the ward nurse, and Dr. Davis, about his patient's IV infusion regimes.

For questions 6 – 10, decide whether each sentence is correct or incorrect. If it is correct, put a tick (√) in the box next to 6 – A for 6 – YES. If it is not correct, put a tick (√) in the box next to 6 – B for 6 – NO. Then mark the corresponding letter on your answer sheet.

You will hear the conversation twice.

Example:

0. Doctor Davis wants to review Mrs. Miles' IV fluids.　　　　**A.** Yes □

B. No ☑

6. Miles is looking after Mrs. Cohen all day today.　　　　**A.** Yes □

B. No □

7. Mrs. Smith's potassium levels are above average.　　　　**A.** Yes □

B. No □

8. Mrs. Smith has been started on one litre of Normal Saline for more than eight hours.

A. Yes ☐

B. No ☐

9. Mrs. Smith's antibiotics are to be given through a separate line.

A. Yes ☐

B. No ☐

10. Mr. Clark's cannula is going to be removed.

A. Yes ☐

B. No ☐

Part 3

Questions 11 – 15

You will hear a conversation between Louisa, the ward nurse, and Gina, about her operation. For questions 11 – 15, choose the correct answer A, B or C. Put a tick (√) in the box. Then mark the corresponding letter on your answer sheet.

You will hear the conversation twice.

11. How is Gina feeling about her coming operation?

A. Very anxious ☐

B. More excited ☐

C. Much confident ☐

12. What kind of operation is she going to have?

A. Transplant surgery ☐

B. Keyhole surgery ☐

C. Emergency surgery ☐

13. The surgeon will carry out the operation with _____.

A. a plastic container ☐

B. a laparoscope ☐

C. a light cover ☐

14. How long will the plastic mini-drain remain inside after the operation?

A. Two or three hours. ☐

B. Three or four days. ☐

C. A week ☐

15. Louisa will ask someone to cover the drain because Gina is _____.

A. afraid of seeing the blood ☐

B. worried about the blood's smell ☐

C. not allowed to see its contents ☐

Part 4

Questions 16 – 20

You will hear a nurse getting personal details from a patient.

Listen and complete questions 16 – 20 on your answer sheet.

You will hear the conversation twice.

Surname Green	First Name (16) _____
Age 42 Sex M	Marital Status M

Occupation Salesman

Present Complaint
(17) _____ chest pain started with severe attack. Pain lasted.
(18) _____ minutes later relieved by rest. Occurred when shopping.

General Condition
RS Chest (19) _____
CVS HR 70/min (20) _____ 130/80
    HS normal

Point to Note
A few more tests should be made.

II. Reading and Writing

Part 1

Questions 21 - 30

Read the descriptions of six cases.

Which case (A-F) mentions this (21-30)? The cases may be chosen more than once. There is an example at the beginning (0).

Mark the correct letter A-F on your answer sheet.

Which case mentions someone who

had his teeth broken?

suffered from loss of hearing?

was weak in the fingers?

had a fever?

suffered from weight loss?

was diagnosed with pericarditis?

lost hair?

could not distinguish hot from cold?

had night sweats?

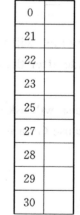

CASE A

Name: James Fox

Age: 6

Occupation: Pupil

Chief complaint: Hit in the face by swing at school.

Other symptoms: Bleeding, no significant fever.

Physical examination: One tooth knocked out, one broken. Missing tooth replaced and splinted. Temporary crown put on broken tooth. No other injuries besides teeth.

CASE B

Name: Art Halamka

Age: 45

Occupation: Housewife

Chief complaint: Chest pain at work.

Other symptoms: Fever.

Physical examination: ECG shows generalized ST segment elevation and there is some pericardial fluid around the heart as shown by echo. The cardiologist diagnosed pericarditis and is going to drain the fluid.

CASE C

Name: Charmine Plantz

Age: 31

Occupation: Sales Manager

Chief complaint: Lump on front of neck for one month.

Other symptoms: Palpitations, heat intolerance, nervousness, insomnia, breathlessness.

Physical examination: Enlarged thyroid. Tachycardia. Slight hypertension. Warm, moist, smooth skin. Exophthalmus. Tremor. Weight loss. Muscle weakness. Hair loss.

CASE D

Name: Selina Burton

Age: 37

Occupation: Typist

Chief complaint: Tingling of first three fingers and thumb that gets worse at night.

Other symptoms: Weakness of fingers (has difficulty buttoning clothes).

Physical examination: Muscle wasting at base of thumb. Unable to distinguish hot from cold.

CASE E

Name: Bob Smithson

Age: 50

Occupation: Construction worker

Chief complaint: Attacks of dizziness with nausea and vomiting. During attack, high pulse rate and rapid breathing. No pattern to attacks.

Other symptoms: Hissing or ringing in ears (on both sides), loss of hearing.

Physical examination: Vital signs normal. Nystagmus. Positive Romberg test.

CASE F

Name: Chuck Talavera

Age: 38

Occupation: Farmer

Chief complaint: Low subjective fever, cough with bad tasting phlegm, night sweats, and weight loss getting worse over the last four months.

Physical examination: Temperature of 38 centigrade, gingival disease, dullness to percussion and absent breath sounds in lower right lobe of lung. Clubbing of fingers.

Part 2

Questions 31 - 40

Read the following passage.

Are sentences 31 - 40 "True" or "False"? If there is not enough information to answer "True" or "False", choose "Not Mentioned". For each sentence (31 - 40), mark one letter A, B or C on your answer sheet.

Being a Nurse Tutor

In Malawi, all hospitals, especially government hospitals, are greatly understaffed. For example, one qualified nurse with the assistance of a patient attendee (similar to the nursing assistants in the UK) looks after a 75-bed tuberculosis ward in a busy city hospital.

Poor pay drives the qualified nurses out of government hospitals to work in the private sector or to take their skills to other countries. Here at St Luke's, we are a mission hospital and it's difficult to keep staff, for similar reasons of a poor wage and allowances package.

I am a nurse tutor and work 50% in the classroom and 50% in the clinical area. My role incorporates the task of teaching in the classroom and also following the students into the clinical area to carry out the teaching of skills, general supervision, and performing assessments of competency. In the UK, tutors very rarely go into the clinical area, as there are always plenty of members of staff to mentor students while they are on their practical placements. This is not the case in Malawi; you will often find students on their own in a ward full of very sick patients.

Through training I try o emphasize the importance of ensuring individualized care, I also stress that nursing is a partnership between the nurse, patient, their friends and family, and that good nursing care is achieved in collaboration with these individuals, and other health professionals in the multi-disciplinary team.

Ensuring that patients are cared for with respect, in a non-judgemental manner, is a very important aspect of my job here in sub-Saharan Africa, where a high percentage of patients in the wards are HIV positive.

I have learnt to cope in a clinical area that is very poorly resourced. I have had to become very inventive and utilize everyday items in an attempt to solve the problems that I come up against. I have also learnt to appreciate the NHS in the UK，and hopefully I will never complain about the lack of resources again!

31. The hospitals in Malawi have plenty of qualified nurses.

    A. True　　　　　　　**B**. False　　　　　　　**C**. Not Mentioned

32. The qualified nurses in Malawi prefer to work in private hospitals.

    A. True　　　　　　　**B**. False　　　　　　　**C**. Not Mentioned

33. Nurse tutors in Malawi need to mentor students in the clinical area.

    A. True　　　　　　　**B**. False　　　　　　　**C**. Not Mentioned

34. Nurse tutors in the UK also supervise the students in the clinical area.

    A. True　　　　　　　**B**. False　　　　　　　**C**. Not Mentioned

35. Nurse students in the UK seldom take care of sick patients on their own in the hospital.

    A. True　　　　　　　**B**. False　　　　　　　**C**. Not Mentioned

36. The writer teaches her students to collaborate with the patients，their friends and family.

    A. True　　　　　　　**B**. False　　　　　　　**C**. Not Mentioned

37. There are many patients who are HIV positive in the suburban London hospitals.

    A. True　　　　　　　**B**. False　　　　　　　**C**. Not Mentioned

38. The writer has had to become inventive in the clinical area in Malawi.

    A. True　　　　　　　**B**. False　　　　　　　**C**. Not Mentioned

39. The clinical area in Malawi is well resourced.

    A. True　　　　　　　**B**. False　　　　　　　**C**. Not Mentioned

40. The qualified nurses are well paid in government hospitals in Malawi.

    A. True　　　　　　　**B**. False　　　　　　　**C**. Not Mentioned

Part 3

Questions 41 – 45

Read the text on the human genome. For questions 41 – 45，choose the answer（A，B or C） which you think fits best according to the text. Mark the correct letter A，B or C on your answer sheet.

Unlocking the Human Genome

A project to unlock secrets—what scientist could resist that challenge? This is what many scientists are doing as they work on the Human Genome Project. The aim of the project is to decode all of the some 100,000 genes in the human body. Scientists are using DNA fingerprinting techniques to do the decoding.

DNA is the substance found in the chromosomes of a cell. A chromosome is a chain of genes. Each gene carries a piece of information. At any one moment in a cell，thousands of genes are turned on and off to produce proteins. The challenge for scientists is to find out what role each gene plays in protein production. At some point this decoding will be complete. Then scientists will have a map of an ideal genome, or a picture of the total genetic nature of a human being. The ideal genome is called a consensus genome. Everything works well in a consensus genome.

But no one in the world has a consensus genome. Everyone's genome is different from the ideal. These differences are referred to as genetic mutations. Genetic mutations in a person's genome mean that the person has a greater than average chance of suffering from health problems. Some problems are not life-threatening. These would include things like baldness, stuttering, or mild headaches. Other problems are serious, such as schizophrenia, heart disease, or diabetes.

The Human Genome Project is one of the most ambitious and challenging quests ever undertaken by science. Its goal is to completely map and sequence all of the genetic material that makes us human. When it is done, we will have a new and profoundly powerful tool to help us to unlock the mysteries of how the human body grows and functions.

41. This passage is mostly about_____ .

   A. how DNA works

   B. decoding all the human genome

   C. the future of science

42. The Human Genome Project is mainly a scientific_____ .

   A. challenge   B. agreement   C. debate

43. When a person's genome is different from the ideal one, the person will probably____
____ .

   A. live much longer than the average people

   B. produce more proteins

   C. suffer from health problems

44. The first sentence in this passage is intended to _____ .

   A. make you angry   B. arouse your interest   C. present the main idea

45. The goal of the Human Genome Project is _____ .

   A. to develop DNA decoding techniques

   B. to identify the role of the ideal genome

   C. to construct a map of the entire human genome

Part 4
Questions 46 – 50

Read the following procedures for skin closure removal. Choose from the procedures A-F the one which fits each gap (46 – 50). There is one extra procedure which you do not need to use. Mark your answers on the answer sheet.

Removal of Skin Closures: Sutures/Staples

Procedure

Ⅰ. Follow the procedure for the aseptic dressing techniques.

Ⅱ. Take care to maintain sterility, open the stitch cutter and forceps or staple remover onto the sterile field.

Ⅲ. (46) _____.

Ⅳ. Wash your hands or use alcohol hand-rub. Make sure that your hands are completely dry before proceeding.

Ⅴ. (47) _____.

Ⅵ. Turn the bag inside out so that the dressing is contained within it, and using the adhesive strip, attach the bag to the side of the trolley or other convenient place close to the wound.

Ⅶ. (48) _____.

Ⅷ. Inspect the wound for signs of healing. If the wound looks inflamed or there is any exudate (pus) present, advice should be sought from an experienced nurse. It may be necessary to remove just one or two sutures/staples to allow the pus to drain.

Ⅸ. Do not clean the wound before removing the sutures/staples, as cleansing solution may seep into the holes made by the sutures/staples when removed.

Ⅹ. (49) _____.

Ⅺ. Use a gauze swab soaked in cleansing solution to clean and then dry around the wound if necessary.

Ⅻ. (50) _____.

ⅩⅢ. If appropriate, apply the new dressing. Remove gloves and discard them into clinical waste bag.

    A. If the wound is longer than 15 cm, remove alternate sutures/staples and check that the wound is fully healed before removing the rest

    B. Open the sterile waste bag and put your hand inside so that the bag acts as a glove. Use this to remove and inspect the old dressing

    C. If there are any small areas where the skin edges are not completely healed together, skin-closure strips may be applied

    D. Adjust any remaining bedclothes to expose the wound; then loosen the existing dressing but do not remove it

    E. Ensure that privacy and dignity are maintained

    F. Take care not to touch the outside of the gloves; put on the sterile gloves

Part 5

Questions 51 – 60

Read the following passage. Choose the best word for each space from a list of words (A-L)

given in the box following the passage. For each space 51 − 60, mark one letter A-L on your answer sheet.

Fresh Sample

It began as a typical working day. As a registered nurse, I traveled to clients' homes to complete paramedical health assessments (51) _____ an insurance company.

As I entered this lady's neat, attractive home, I smelled the delicious aroma of pies (52) _____."Umm, sure smells good in here, " I commented.

"I just put a couple of lemon meringue pies (53) _____ the oven. They're my husband's favorite, " my client volunteered.

Returning to the purpose of my visit, we (54) _____ the questionnaire quickly. The last section involved collecting a urine sample.

"I collected it earlier (55) _____ saved it in the refrigerator, " she said. "I'll get if for you."

(56) _____ I emptied the sample into the collection tubes, I noticed the unusual thickness of it. When I tested it with a dip stick, I was (57) _____ at the extremely high protein content.

" Are you sure this is your urine sample?" I questioned. "(58) _____ almost resembles egg whites. "

"Yes, I distinctly remember placing it in the refrigerator in the bottom right-hand corner. Oh! Oh, no!" She wailed. "I've made a terrible mistake. Don't use that. I'll (59) _____ you a fresh sample. "

Not wishing to further embarrass the lady, I asked no more questions. But as I opened the door to leave her home, I (60) _____ her removing pies from the oven and the grinding sound of the garbage disposal.

No lemon meringue pie that night!

A. heard	**B.** for	**C.** get	**D.** these
E. As	**F.** shocked	**G.** send	**H.** in
I. and	**J.** completed	**K.** baking	**L.** It

Part 6

Question 61

Read the patient's discharge summary.

Use the information in the summary to write a report.

*Write the report in about **100 words** on your answer sheet.*

DISCHARGE SUMMARY

Patient Mrs. Martha	**Date of Birth** 17/09/1938
Date of Discharge 10 May, 2015	**Date of Admission** 23 April, 2015

Problems
- Has been suffering from hypertension & degenerative bone disease
- Needs to urinate frequently
- Diagnosed with pneumonia & urinary tract infection

Next of Kin
- No immediate family

Needs
- Bath seat and safety rails in bathroom
- Nurse to visit twice per week to monitor medications
- Physiotherapy three times per week

Strengths and Resources
- Independent-minded woman, fully alert and articulate, can cook

METS(二级)样卷(B)

医护英语水平考试

(二级)

Medical English Test System(METS)

Level 2

姓名_____   准考证号_____   时间：120 分钟

考生注意事项

1. 严格遵守考场规则,考生得到监考人员的指令后方可开始答题。
2. 考生须将自己的姓名和准考证号写在本试卷上。
3. 作答前,考生务必将自己的姓名、准考证号用黑色字迹的签字笔填写在答题卡指定位置,并将准考证号对应的信息点用 2B 铅笔涂黑。
4. 全部试题均在答题卡上作答,在试卷上作答无效。选择题部分,用 2B 铅笔把答题卡上对应题目的答案标号涂黑。如需改动,用橡皮擦干净后,再涂选其他答案。非选择题部分,用黑色字迹的签字笔在答题卡的指定位置答题。
5. 考试结束后考生将试题和答题卡放在桌上,不得带走,待监考人员收毕清点后,方可离场。任何个人或机构不得保留、复制和出版本试卷,不得以任何形式传播试卷内容。违者必究。

教育部考试中心

××××年××月

Ⅰ. Listening

Part 1

Questions 1 – 5

You will hear five patients complaining their sufferings to the nurse. What does each patient complain of? For questions 1 – 5, mark the correct letter A-H on your answer sheet. You will hear each conversation twice.

Example:

0. Wood

0	A	B	C	D	E	F	G	H
	☐	☐	☐	☐	☐	■	☐	☐

1. Hales   **A.** Headache
2. Lan   **B.** Shortness of breath
3. Jack   **C.** Cough
4. Swift   **D.** Pain in the chest
5. Bloomfield   **E.** High temperature

                        F. Pain in the hands

                        G. Dizziness

                        H. Sore throat

Part 2

Questions 6 – 10

You will hear a conversation between Sophie, the ward nurse, and Mr. Jones, the patient, about wound management.

For questions 6 – 10, decide whether each sentence is correct or incorrect.

If it is correct, put a tick (√) in the box next to A for YES. If it is not correct, put a tick (√) in the box next to B for NO. Then mark the corresponding letter on your answer sheet. You will hear the conversation twice.

Example:

0. Sophie is the wound management Clinical Nurse Specialist.   **A.** Yes ☑

                                                            B. No ☐

6. Mr. Jones rejected Sophie's request of having a quick look at his leg wound.

                                                            A. Yes ☐

                                                            B. No ☐

7. Mr. Jones has been managing quite well at home.   **A.** Yes ☐

                                                            B. No ☐

8. Sophie thinks the first thing to do is to reassess the wound. **A.** Yes ☐
   B. No ☐

9. A VAC is a type of dressing method different from the previous one. **A.** Yes ☐
   B. No ☐

10. Mr. Jones' wound is expected to heal faster. **A.** Yes ☐
    B. No ☐

Part 3

Questions 11 – 15

You will hear a conversation between Helen, the ward nurse, and Mr. Albiston, about his new medication, atorvastatin（阿托伐他汀）. For questions 11 – 15, choose the correct answer A, B or C. Put a tick（√）in the box. Then mark the corresponding letter on your answer sheet. You will hear the conversation twice.

11. How often should atorvastatin be taken? **A.** Once a day ☐
    B. Twice a day ☐
    C. Three times a day ☐

12. Atorvastatin works _____. **A.** quite quickly ☐
    B. quite slowly ☐
    C. just so-so ☐

13. Atorvastatin is metabolized, or chemically changed _____.
    A. in the stomach ☐
    B. in the small intestines ☐
    C. in the liver ☐

14. Atorvastatin is used for patients with high levels of _____.
    A. "good" cholesterol ☐
    B. "bad" cholesterol ☐
    C. "good" and "bad" cholesterol ☐

15. What time of day is atorvastatin suggested to be taken?
    A. in the morning ☐
    B. in the afternoon ☐
    C. in the evening ☐

Part 4

Questions 16 – 20

You will hear a nurse getting personal details from a patient.
Listen and complete questions 16 – 20 on your answer sheet.
You will hear the conversation twice.

Surname Connolly	First Name (16) _____

D. O. B (17) _____ Sex M	Marital Status M

Hospital Number (18) _____

Clinical Impression Asthma

Allergies (19) _____

General Condition
O/E:
CVS HR 64/min (20) _____ 130/80
HS normal

II. Reading and Writing

Part 1

Questions 21 – 30

Read the descriptions of six cases. Which case(A-F) mentions this (21 – 30)? The cases may be chosen more than once. There is an example at the beginning (0). Mark the correct letter A-F on your answer sheet.

Which case mentions someone who

was constipated?

suffered from tremor of the right hand?

was sleeping poorly?

had a weight change?

suffered from tiredness?

had a normal pregnancy at age 25?

lost hair?

complained of swelling ankles?

had a painless lump on the right side of the neck?

0	
21	
22	
23	
25	
27	
28	
29	
30	

24	
26	

CASE A

A 50-year-old housewife，who had been well until four months previously，complained of tiredness and malaise (不舒服). She had gained 9kg in weight in the year before she presented to her GP although she denied eating more than usual. She was constipated and she noticed that her hair had started to fall out.

CASE B

A 33-year-old man presented to his GP complaining of a painless lump on the right side of his neck, which had been present for about two months and was enlarging. He had been feeling generally unwell and had lost about 5kg in weight. He was also complaining of night sweats. He had no significant past medical history.

CASE C

On examination, her face showed little or no expression. There was a tremor affecting mainly her right hand. She had generally increased muscle tone. Power, reflexes (反应), coordination and sensation were within normal limits. Examination of her gait (步态) showed that she was slow to start walking and had difficulty in stopping and turning.

CASE D

A 56-year-old woman presented to her GP, complaining of increased tiredness over the past few months. She had lost interest in most things. She was sleeping poorly and tended to wake up early, but denied any suicidal tendencies. She was thirsty and was passing urine more often. She was eating normally and her weight was steady.

CASE E

A 60-year-old man attended his GP's surgery, complaining of breathlessness on exertion. This had been increasing over the previous eight months until it was producing problems at around 500 meters walking on the level. There was no history of chest pain. He had noticed some swelling ankles by the end of the day. This disappeared overnight.

CASE F

A 45-year-old woman had been having prolonged periods lasting for 8 days, with the passage of clots for 9 months. There was no bleeding between periods or after intercourse. Her periods were not particularly painful. She had not noticed any hot flushes or night sweats and her general health had always been good. She had had a normal pregnancy when she was 25.

Part 2

Questions 31 - 40

Read the following passage. Are sentences 31 - 40 "True" or "False"? If there is not enough information to answer "True" or "False", choose "Not Mentioned". For each sentence (31 - 40), mark one letter A, B or C on your answer sheet.

Pre-operative Assessment

At the pre-operative assessment it is important to check that the patient is fit for surgery. This is especially so as many of the patients are elderly and may have other health problems. Common conditions like high blood pressure and diabetes need to be adequately controlled before the cataract operation can safely proceed. If the patient is taking an anticoagulant(阻凝剂),e.g. warfarin(华法林阻凝剂)，the blood clotting may need to be checked and the dose of the drug adjusted，in liaison with the patient's general practitioner or haematologist(血液病专家).

If the operation is to be under local anaesthetic，the assessor should check that the patient can lie reasonably flat and still without undue distress for as long as the surgery will take，typically about 15 – 20 minutes.

If a general anaesthetic is planned，then some additional investigations may be needed，e. g. an EGG (electrocardiogram) and perhaps some simple blood tests，and these can be organized at the pre-operative assessment. If the patient has significant heart or breathing problems，then the anaesthetist may wish to examine the patient before the day of surgery. As a general rule，a cataract operation，even under a local anaesthetic，should not be performed within 3 months of a heart attack or stroke. This is because even though the surgery itself may not unduly disturb the general health of the patient，it is nonetheless a stressful experience for some.

For example，the worry and anxiety of the ordeal(折磨) may increase blood pressure which could place an undue strain on a recently damaged heart or circulatory system. Opinions on the length of rehabilitation before surgery may differ a little between specialists and some may feel that a longer period is wise，particularly if a general anaesthetic is contemplated (考虑).

31. Pre-operative assessment is performed in order to find out whether patients are unsuitable candidates of the operation.

    A. True   **B**. False   **C**. Not Mentioned

32. According to the passage，the health checks are prepared only for patients who are elderly or who have some medical problems.

    A. True   **B**. False   **C**. Not Mentioned

33. Pre-operative assessment has a universal format.

    A. True   **B**. False   **C**. Not Mentioned

34. The surgery will usually take about 15 – 20 minutes.

    A. True   **B**. False   **C**. Not Mentioned

35. Patients who have significant heart or breathing problems should do some simple blood tests before the day of surgery.

    A. True   **B**. False   **C**. Not Mentioned

36. A cataract operation can be arranged within 3 months of a heart attack.

    A. True   **B**. False   **C**. Not Mentioned

37. For some patients，a surgery brings about worries and anxieties.

    A. True   **B**. False   **C**. Not Mentioned

38. At the pre-operative assessment，psychological consultation can also be provided to the patient.

A. True   B. False   C. Not Mentioned

39. It may be wise to plan a lengthy period of rehabilitation before the patient is operated on.

A. True   B. False   C. Not Mentioned

40. A general anaesthetic is more recommendable than a local one.

A. True   B. False   C. Not Mentioned

Part 3

Questions 41 – 45

Read the following text on first aid. For questions 41 – 45, choose the answer (A, B or C) which you think fits best according to the text. Mark the correct letter A, B or C on your answer sheet.

First Aid

First aid is emergency care for a victim of sudden illness or injury until more skillful medical treatment is available. It may save a life or improve certain vital signs including pulse, temperature, a clear airway, and breathing. In minor emergencies, first aid may prevent a victim's condition from turning worse and provide relief from pain. First aid must be administered as quickly as possible. In the case of the critically injured, a few minutes can make the difference between complete recovery and loss of life.

First-aid measures depend upon a victim's needs and the provider's level of knowledge and skill. Knowing what not to do in an emergency is as important as knowing what to do. Improperly moving a person with a neck injury, for example, can lead to permanent spinal injury and paralysis.

Despite the variety of possible injures, several principle of first aid apply to all emergencies. The first step is to call for professional medical help. The victim, if conscious, should be reassured that medical aid has been requested, and asked for permission to provide any first aid. Next, assess the scene, asking other people or the injured person's family or friends about details of the injury or illness, any care that may have already been given, and preexisting conditions such as diabetes or heart trouble. The victim should be checked for a medical bracelet or card that describes special medical conditions. Unless the accident scene becomes unsafe or the victim may suffer further injury, do not move the victim.

First aid requires rapid assessment of victims to determine whether life-threatening conditions exist. One method for evaluating a victim's condition is known by the acronym (首字母缩写词) ABC, which stands for:

A-irway: Is it open and clear?

B-reathing: Is the person breathing? Look, listen, and feel for breathing.

C-irculation: Is there a pulse? Is the person bleeding externally? Check skin color and temperature for additional indications of circulation problems.

41. First aid may bring about all the following results EXCEPT _____ .

    A. relieving a victim from pain

    B. preventing a victim's condition from getting worse

    C. helping a person avoid sudden illness or injury

42. Before we administer first aid to a victim，it is very important for us _____ .

    A. to refer to all kinds of handbooks on first aid

    B. to make sure what to do and what not to do

    C. to remove the ring or bracelet he may be wearing

43. In administering first aid to a victim，you should first of all _____ .

    A. Turn him over

    B. remove him from the accident scene

    C. Call for professional medical help

44. You may assess a victim's condition by all the following EXCEPT _____ .

    A. checking whether there is a pulse

    B. replacing his medical bracelet or card

    C. looking，listening and feeling for breathing

45. The purpose of the passage is to tell the reader _____ .

    A. some basic facts about first aid

    B. the important of protecting the accident

    C. what professional medical help is

Part 4

Questions 46 – 50

Read the following procedures for administering intramuscular injection. Choose from the procedures A-F the one which fits each gap(46 –50). There is one extra procedure which you do not need to use. Mark your answers on the answer sheet.

Administering Intramuscular Injection

Procedure

Ⅰ. Check the medication order.

Ⅱ. (46) _____ .

Ⅲ. If the medication is particularly irritating to subcutaneous tissue，change the needle on the syringe before the injection.

Ⅳ. (47) _____ .

Ⅴ. Establish the exact site for the injection and assist the patient to an appropriate position，usually the patient should be prone，with his toes pointed inward.

Ⅵ. (48) _____ .

Ⅶ. Remove the needle cover.

Ⅷ. Push the syringe and expel any excess air that accidentally entered the syringe.

Ⅸ. Use the non-dominant hand to spread the skin at the site.

Ⅹ. (49) _____ .

Ⅺ. Aspirate(吸出) by holding the barrel of the syringe steady with your non-dominant hand and by pulling back on the plunger with your dominant hand. If blood appears in the syringe, withdraw the needle, discard the syringe, and prepare a new injection. If blood dose does not appear, inject the medication steadily and slowly, holding the syringe steady.

Ⅻ. (50) _____ .

ⅩⅢ. Dispose of materials, wash your hands, chart the injection, and observe the patient.

    A. Clear the site with an antiseptic swab. Using a circular motion, start at the center and move outward about 5 cm

    B. Select the intramuscular site for adequate muscular mass

    C. Ensure privacy and dignity

    D. Holding the syringe between the thumb and forefinger, pierce the skin quickly at a 90 degree angle, and insert the needle into the muscle

    E. Following the injection, the site is massaged thoroughly to promote absorption

    F. Prepare the correct dosage of the drug from a vial or an ampule

Part 5

Questions 51 – 60

Read the following passage. Choose the best word for each space from a list of words (A-L) given in the box following the passage. For each space 51 – 60, mark one letter A-L on your answer sheet.

Ways to Prevent Osteoporosis

Even if you feel as strong as an ox, you may still be at risk for osteoporosis. This condition develops when your bones lose mass and density, (51) _____ them to become porous(多孔的), weak and brittle(脆的). As the bones weaken, they become more (52) _____ to fractures that can cause serious health consequences.

Although osteoporosis tends to affect older people—especially women after menopause—you can lower the risk of this disease significantly (53) _____ taking certain actions when you are younger.

Perform weight-bearing exercise. The risk of osteoporosis for both men and women depends largely on the (54) _____ of bone mass attained between the age of 25 and 35. Developing a peak store of bone mass will help protect you when your bones(55) _____ begin to thin. Weight-bearing exercise is one of the best ways to increase bone mass because bone responds to exercise by becoming denser. (56) _____ it is important to build as much bone mass as possible when you are younger, exercise at all ages helps the bones. Examples of weight-bearing activities include lifting weights, walking or running, tennis, and dancing.

Get adequate(57) _____ of calcium and vitamin D. Eating foods high in calcium helps strengthen bones. Obtaining adequate levels of calcium is particularly important while the skeleton is growing in childhood and adolescence and during pregnancy and breastfeeding. (58) _____ sufficient level of vitamin D is also crucial to keeping bones healthy because this mineral is essential for helping the body to absorb calcium.

Do not smoke. Smoking increases bone loss, although scientists aren't exactly sure why. Many experts believe this (59) _____ because smoking decreases a woman's production of estrogen and reduces the absorption of calcium in the intestine. It is not known whether or not (60) _____ to secondhand smoke can affect a person's bone mass.

A. amount	B. exposure	C. causing	D. content
E. inevitably	F. Consuming	G. Since	H. intake
I. susceptible	J. Although	K. occurs	L. by

Part 6

Question 61

Read the following medical note.

*Use the note to write a case report in about **100 words** on your answer sheet.*

MEDICAL NOTE	
Patient Mr. Martha	**Age** 36
Date of Discharge 10 May, 2015	**Date of Admission** 23 April, 2015

Reason for Admission
- Review of a venous ulcer

Past Medical History
- IDDM (insulin-dependent diabetes mellitus)
- HT (hypertension)
- MI (myocardial infarction) four months ago

Past Surgical History
- Femoral-popliteal bypass four months ago

Medication
- Insulin, half an aspirin and a multivitamin

Allergies
- Penicillin and codeine (可待因)

Next of Kin
- No immediate family

METS(二级)答题卡

医护英语水平考试二级答题卡

MEDICAL ENGLISH TEST SYSTEM (METS) LEVEL 2

姓名

有效填涂

无效填涂

准考证号

填涂要求

1. 答题前，考生务必用黑色字迹笔在答题卡上填写清楚姓名、准考证号，书写准考证号时一格一位数字，从左往右依次填写，核对无误后使用2B铅笔把每一位准考证号对应的标号涂黑。
2. 选择题必须用2B铅笔按照示例的正确方法填涂，修改时要用橡皮擦干净，其它题目必须用黑色字迹笔书写。
3. 答题时注意题号顺序。
4. 保持答题卡的清洁和完整，不得折叠。

填涂示例

缺考违纪标记栏

缺考   违纪

I Listening

II Reading and Writing

III Write your answer below

(请在背面答题区作答)

61.

参考答案

Unit 1
Part I
Topic-related Terms
1. b 2. a 3. c 4. e 5. d
Text Exploration
1. T 2. F 3. T 4. T 5. F
Part III
Critical Thinking
1. Data is gathered about the patient, family or community that the nurse is working with. Objective data, or data that can be collected through examination, is measurable. This includes things like vital signs or observable patient behaviors. Subjective data is gathered from patients as they talk about their needs, feelings and perspectives about the problems they're having.
2. To take the medicine and do some exercises.
3. The nursing process is the systematic method of assessing, diagnosing, planning, implementing and evaluating nursing care. It plays an very important role in the nurse's approach. It's the method used by nurses to solve clients' problems. It is the basis of nursing practice. It can help a nurse to use time and resources effectively and help nurses to clarify their responsibility and nursing standards.
4. Medical diagnosis is a noun used by doctors to determine a specific disease or pathological condition. It's the judgment of the patient's health and the nature of the disease. The number of medical diagnoses is relatively small and relatively stable in the course of disease development. Within the scope of the doctor's responsibility, doctors prescribe prescriptions for prevention and treatment. Nurses perform physician orders and monitor the development of the disease. On the means of medical diagnosis, medical measures and nursing measures are both used. Nursing diagnosis is a noun used by nurses to judge the reactions of individuals or groups to existing or potential health problems or diseases. The number of nursing diagnoses is varied and varies with the patient's response. With the scope of care, nurses are required to conduct independent care and preventive and curative work. Through the care measures problems can be resolved independently.

Unit 2
Part I
Topic-related Terms
1. f 2. e 3. g 4. h 5. c 6. d 7. a 8. b

Text Exploration

1. T 2. F 3. F 4. T 5. F

Part Ⅲ

Critical Thinking

1. (1) Warmly welcomes the patient.

    (2) Introduces the hospital.

    (3) Fills in the inpatient medical record, hospitalization list card and bedside card.

    (4) Completes a physical examination.

    (5) Tells the doctor to view the patient.

    (6) Completes the first nursing record and communicates with the patient.

    (7) The head nurse greets and introduces herself to the patients.

2. The reasons are as follows:

    (1) Help patients ease the anxiety of just entering the hospital.

    (2) Better understand the personality, physiological state and needs of the patient and make good preparation for the doctor to implement targeted treatment.

3. The physical examinations which patients should take before admission are as follows:
   body temperature, pulse, respiration, blood pressure, weight, etc.

   Reason:

   The above examination is not only for the doctor to fully understand the physical condition of the patient, but also for the requirements of each hospital, and is responsible for the patients.

4. In order to serve our patients, as a nurse, I should do the following:

    (1) have skillful nursing skills;

    (2) have a good cautious independence;

    (3) maintain good work mood;

    (4) have team spirit;

    (5) strengthen basic knowledge and improve professional ability;

    (6) have good service attitude and communication skills.

Unit 3

Part Ⅰ

Topic-related Terms

1. c 2. f 3. e 4. h 5. i 6. b 7. a 8. d 9. a 10. g

Text Exploration

1. F 2. F 3. F 4. T 5. T

Part Ⅲ

Critical Thinking

1. It is necessary to remove the patient's sleeve and expose the area of the brachial artery in case the blood would not flow smoothly and thus the BP result would be affected.

2. It can be distinguished in this way: the first voice of the brachial pulse heard is systolic pressure and the hanged voice or disappearance of the brachial pulse heard is diastolic pressure.

3. The purpose is to keep mercury down slowly enough and get a correct BP result. If expel the air too slowly, it will cause venous congestion and make the diastolic pressure higher. If expel the air too fast, the changes of voice of systolic pressure and diastolic pressure cannot be detected clearly.

4. Re-measure the blood pressure or get the mini-value from 2 to 3 continuous measurement.

Unit 4

Part I

Topic-related Terms

1. g 2. h 3. c 4. a 5. b 6. e 7. f 8. d

Text Exploration

1. T 2. T 3. F 4. F 5. T

Part III

Critical Thinking

1. In order to prevent the occurrence of anaphylaxis, especially the occurrence of severe allergic reactions, it is required that the skin sensitivity test should be done before use of penicillin. Skin test negative drugs can be used for patients, and skin test positive drugs are prohibited.

2. In the clinical use of penicillin, there are more anaphylaxis, including rash, drug fever, vascular neurodropsy, serological type reaction, anaphylactic shock and so on. These are known as penicillins anaphylaxis, and allergic shock is the most serious. Anaphylactic shock occurs more than a few minutes after the injection. Symptoms are dyspnea, cyanosis, blood pressure drop, coma, ankylosis, and final convulsion. The patient can die within a short time..

3. If you have taken penicillin without realizing you have an allergy, stop taking it. Then, your doctor may prescribe a medicine called an antihistamine, such as diphenhydramine, to help with your symptoms. For more serious problems such as swelling, she might give you a medicine called a corticosteroid. With anaphylaxis, she may give you a drug called epinephrine right away. You'll spend some time in the hospital until your blood pressure and breathing are better.

4. When you can't take penicillin, you normally avoid it. Your doctor will try to find another kind of antibiotic. If you really need penicillin, you may get a treatment called desensitization. You usually would get this only if you didn't react with anaphylaxis previously. In desensitization, your doctor will start you with a small dose of penicillin. If you don't show allergy symptoms in 15 to 30 minutes, then you get a higher dose. You get higher doses over a few hours or days. If you don't have symptoms, then you can keep taking penicillin.

Unit 5

Part I

Topic-related Terms

1. d 2. g 3. a 4. f 5. b 6. h 7. c 8. e

Text Exploration

1. T 2. F 3. F 4. F 5. T

Part III

Critical Thinking

1. First, finding the most appropriate position for the patient based on age and ability to co-operate. Second, check the tube whether it is intact. The length for the infant and children is from the bridge of the nose to the ear lobe, then from the ear lobe to xiphisternum. While for neonates is from the nose to ear and then to the halfway point between xiphisternum and

umbilicus. Third，bending the patient's head slightly forward and gently pass the tube into the patient's nostril，advancing it along the floor of the nasopharynx to the oropharynx. Never advance the tube against resistance. If the patient shows signs of breathlessness or severe coughing，remove the tube immediately. Lastly，lightly secure the tube with tape，or have an assistant hold the tube in place until the position has been checked.

2. Nurse should gather together all the equipment needed such as appropriate size and type of tube，sterile water，foil bowl and tissues，pH indicator paper，20 ml syringe，non-sterile gloves，tape and place on a clean tray. And then wash and dry hands thoroughly，put on non-sterile gloves and apron.

3. The most appropriate position for the patient depends on age and ability to co-operate.

4. Stop advancing the tube against resistance.

Unit 6

Part Ⅰ

Topic-related Terms

1. b 2. e 3. a 4. c 5. d

Text Exploration

1. T 2. T 3. F 4. T 5. T

Part Ⅲ

Critical Thinking

1. Indications for suprapubic catheterization：

   (1) urethra trauma；

   (2) clients who require long-term catheterization and who are sexually active；

   (3) following pelvic or urological surgery；

   (4) some gynaecological conditions，e.g. colposuspension；

   (5) long-term catheterization for incontinence；

   (6) clients who are unable to tolerate urethral catheterization；

   (7) some wheelchair-bound clients.

2. Factors influencing urination：

   1) psychological factors：anxiety and emotional stress ；emotional tension；heard sound of running water；

   2) personal habits；

   3) sociocultural factors；

   4) volume status：ingestion of certain fluids directly affects urine production and excretion；

   5) climate changes：

      (1) in summer：urine production decreasing；

      (2) in winter：urine production increasing. ；

   6) treatment and checking：the clients often lose blood in the operation thus lead to decrease the urine excretion；

   7) disease conditions：

      (1) any lesion of peripheral nerves leads to reduce sensation of bladder fullness，and difficulty in controlling urination. For example，diabetes mellitus can alter bladder function；

      (2) diseases that hinder physical activity interfere with the ability to void. For example，a

client with rheumatoid arthritis often cannot sit on or rise from a toilet without an elevated seat;

(3) and diseases damage to the glomerulus or tubules can also influence the urination.

8) growth and development.

3. Indications for use of urinary catheters:

1) short-term catheterization:

(1) urologic surgery;

(2) surgery on contiguous structures;

(3) critically ill patients requiring accurate measure of urinary output;

(4) acute urinary retention;

2) long-term catheterization:

(1) bladder outlet obstruction not correctable medical or surgically;

(2) intractable skin breakdown caused or exacerbated by incontinence;

(3) some patients with neurogenic bladder and retention;

(4) palliative care for terminally ill or severely impaired incontinent patients for whom bed and clothing changes are uncomfortable;

(5) preference of a patient who has not responded to specific incontinence treatments ;

4. Guidelines for prevention of Catheter-Associated UTI:

1) category 1. strongly recommended:

(1) catheterize only when necessary;

(2) educate personnel in correct techniques of catheter insertion and care;

(3) emphasize handwashing;

(4) insert catheter using aseptic technique and sterile equipment;

(5) secure catheter properly;

(6) maintain closed sterile drainage;

(7) obtain urine specimens aseptically;

(8) maintain unobstructed urine flow;

2) category 2. moderately recommended:

(1) periodically re-educate personnel in catheter care;

(2) use smallest suitable catheter bore;

(3) avoid irrigation unless needed to prevent or relieve obstruction;

(4) refrain from daily meatal care.

(5) do not change catheters at arbitrary intervals.

Unit 7
Part I
Topic-related Terms
1. f 2. e 3. d 4. b 5. g 6. c 7. h 8. a
Text Exploration
1. T 2. T 3. F 4. T 5. F
Part III
Critical Thinking
1. Aseptic techniques in health care are important to keep infectious microorganisms from sterile surfaces or tissues. In health care aseptic techniques deter infection when working with

patients.

2. 1) The surroundings should be clean.

   2) Doctor and nurse should put on uniform round cap, shoes and mask. Fail nails short and wash hands before aseptic procedures. Wear sterile gloves if it is necessary.

   3) Maintenance of aseptic supply:

   (1) place aseptic articles and non-aseptic articles separately;

   (2) keep aseptic articles in sterile containers or sterile packages;

   (3) once taken out of the container or package, aseptic article can't be put back even having never been used;

   (4) there is a label (with the name and sterile date) on the container or package. Expiration date is 7 days. If it comes to the expiry date or the package is wet, re-sterilize it.

   4) Applying aseptic technique correctly:

   (1) keep away from the aseptic field (about 20 – 30 cm) during procedures;

   (2) use sterile transfer forceps or tissue forceps to fetch sterile item;

   (3) keep hands, arms and sterile item above the waist level;

   (4) do not touch sterile item or field with non-sterile item, hand or forearm;

   (5) do not reach across sterile field;

   (6) non-sterile item or potential contaminated item is inhibited during aseptic procedures;

   (7) a set of aseptic supply is only used once upon a client.

3. 1) Applying sterile transfer forceps.

   2) Applying sterile container.

   3) Using sterile package.

   4) Preparing sterile therapeutic tray.

   5) Pouring sterile solution.

   6) Donning and taking off sterile gloves.

4. 1) Once a package has been opened, the remaining items need to be used within 24 hours.

   2) If the items are contaminated or the wrapper is wet, re-sterilize them.

Unit 8

Part I

Topic-related Terms

1. a 2. d 3. e 4. b 5. c 6. f 7. h 8. g

Text Exploration

1. T 2. T 3. F 4. F 5. T

Part III

Critical Thinking

1. (1) To decrease shortness of breath and fatigue (tiredness).

   (2) To improve sleep in some people who have sleep-related breathing disorders.

   (3) To improve the lifespan of some people who have COPD.

2. Abide by the regulations of the procedure strictly. Pay attention to the safety of administering oxygen. "Four preventions" (including fire prevention, quake prevention, hot prevention and oil prevention) are fulfilled. Avoid shaking the oxygen cylinder to escape exploding. The oxygen cylinder should be placed in the shade. Forbid placing the pyrotechnical and tinderbox near the oxygen cylinder. Move the stove from the oxygen cylinder about 5 meters, and from a

radiator about 1 meter. Tell the patient and the family not to smoke in the ward. Avoid using oil towel in the ward, even screwing the safety value using hands with oil. Oil can ignite spontaneously in the presence of oxygen.

3. No smoking here. Don't adjust the flow rate by yourself, it's a dangerous thing.

4. Assess the change of patient's pulse, blood pressure, the state of consciousness, the color and the temperature of skin, the respiratory mode during the oxygen therapy, which can scale the effects of the oxygen therapy. Mensurating the Arterial Blood Gases (ABG) can help to assess the effects and select the appropriate rate of flow.

Unit 9

Part I

Topic-related Terms

1. c 2. e 3. a 4. g 5. f 6. d 7. h 8. b

Text Exploration

1. F 2. T 3. F 4. T 5. T

Part III

Critical Thinking

1. I think they should be as strong as possible since it is probably necessary for them to carry the heavy patient into or out of the wheelchair and then into the car.

2. First, adjustments of the wheelchair should be made. That's to say, when elevating the patient just off the surface, the nurses must check again to make sure the sling is properly adjusted and connected to the studs on the arms. If any attachments are not properly in place, immediately lower the patient back onto the surface and correct this problem. Second, the transfer should be made on the level driveway or the surface.

3. By explaining clearly to the patient the procedure and the importance of cooperation and by showing them how to do it.

4. Yes, I think I can. To do the work well, I will first get a good idea of the patient. Then I will make good preparation for it in advance. Finally, I'll operate it carefully according to standards and the procedures concerned.

METS(二级)样卷(A)

I. Listening

Part 1 1. B 2. D 3. H 4. G 5. E

Part 2 6. B 7. B 8. B 9. A 10. A

Part 3 11. A 12. B 13. B 14. A 15. A

Part 4 16. Peter 17. Central 18. 10 19. clear 20. BP/Blood Pressure

II. Reading and Writing

Part 1

21. E 查找：other symptoms：...loss of hearing

22. D 查找：other symptoms：weakness of fingers...

23. B 查找：other symptoms：fever

24. F 查找：chief complaint：Low subjective fever...

25. C 查找：physical examination：Weight loss

26. F 查找：chief complaint：...and weight loss getting worse

27. B 查找：physical examination：The cardiologist diagnosed pericarditis...

28. C 查找：physical examination：Hair loss

29. D 查找：physical examination：Unable to distinguish hot from cold

30. F 查找：chief complaint：...night sweats...

Part 2

文章大意：本文介绍一位护理学教师在非洲马拉维的工作情况、她对学生的要求，以及她如何应对工作中的各种困难。

31. B 从句首"In Malawi, all hospitals, especially government hospitals, are greatly understaffed."判断，应该是人员不足。

32. A 参见第二段"Poor pay drives the qualified nurses out of government hospitals to work in the private sector or to take their skills to other countries."

33. A 参见第三段"I am a nurse tutor and work 50% in the classroom and 50% in the clinical area."

34. B 参见第三段"In the UK, tutors very rarely go into the clinical area, as there are always plenty of members of staff to mentor students while they are on their practical placements."

35. A 参见第三段"there are always plenty of members of staff to mentor students while they are on their practical placements. This is not the case in Malawi; you will often find students on their own in a ward full of very sick patients."

36. A 参见第四段。

37. C 参见第五段，文章只提到非洲撒哈拉以南地区，未涉及英国 HIV 的病人。

38. A 参见最后一段"I have also learnt to appreciate the NHS in the UK, and hopefully I will never complain about the lack of resources again!"

39. B 从最后一段第一句判断哪儿应该是资源匮乏，而非丰富。

40. B 从第二段第一句判断，马拉维政府医院合格护士报酬很低。

Part 3

文章大意：本文介绍了人类基因组解密研究计划，涉及不少术语，如 DNA、染色体、细胞、基因、蛋白质合成、理想基因组、基因突变等。

41. B 考查文章的主题。从标题、第一段与尾段判断，本文主要是介绍解密人类基因组计划。Unlock 与 decode 同义。

42. A 人类基因组计划是一项科学挑战。第一段第一句、第二段第五句以及第四段第一句分别出现了 challenge 和 challenging。

43. C 当个人的基因与理性基因组不同时，这个人可能出现健康问题。

44. B 解读文章第一句话的写作意图，主要是引发读者的兴趣。

45. C 人类基因组计划的研究目标是构建一幅完整的人类蓝图。参见尾段第二句"Its goal is to completely map and sequence all of the genetic material that makes us human. material that makes us human."

Part 4

46. D 47. B 48. F 49. A 50. C

文章大意：本文介绍了拆线和拆肘钉的步骤。

一、遵守无菌换药技术。

二、注意保持无菌，打开拆线刀镊子或是起钉器。

三、调整好病人衣物以便露出伤口，松开敷料，但不要移除。

101

四、洗手或使用酒精擦手。操作前确保两手完全干燥。

五、打开无菌污物袋，将手放到里面，这样袋子就可充当手套，然后小心去除敷料。

六、将袋子外翻，包住敷料，使用胶布把袋子粘在旁边的手推车上或其他靠近伤口的便利位置。

七、戴上无菌手套，注意不要碰触到手套外部。

八、检查伤口愈合情况。如果伤口发炎了或有脓液，应该咨询有经验的护士。此时只需拆除一两处缝线或肘钉，以便脓液引流。

九、移除缝线或肘钉前不要清洗伤口，因为清洗液可能渗入移除缝线或肘钉时造成的小孔中。

十、如果伤口超过 15 厘米，交替移除缝线或肘钉，在移除剩余缝线或肘钉前检查伤口是否完全愈合。

十一、如有必要，使用浸过清洗液的纱布清洗伤口，然后擦干。

十二、如果出现小范围皮肤边缘未完全愈合，可以使用胶布。

十三、如果需要，重新更换敷料，结束后脱下手套丢到医疗垃圾袋中。

Part 5

文章大意：文中护士为保险公司到客户家完成健康评估，结果该客户把事先准备的尿液样本当成甜饼佐料用来烤甜饼了。

51．B　文中护士是为一家保险公司去完成对客户的健康评估，故选择 for。

52．K　烤甜饼表示当时正在进行。

53．H　(甜饼)放到烤箱里烤。

54．J　完成问卷调查。

55．I　此处表示前后事件的承接。

56．E　按照该句前后意义关系，此处为时间状语从句，意思是"当……时"。

57．F　根据后面的"the extremely high protein content"，此处表示"吃惊"。

58．L　根据前后意义关系，此处指代 the urine sample，故用 it。

59．C　此处表示"让你得到"之意，因为该尿液样本是需要交给护士检查的。

60．A　此处表示作者打开门要离开时"听到"声音，后面的 and the grinding sound 也起到提示作用。

Part 6

参考样文：

Discharge Summary

Mrs. Martha was born on 17 September, 1938. She was admitted on 23 April, 2015, and discharge on 10 May, 2015.

There are still some problems to be solved after discharge. For example, she has been suffering from hypertension and degenerative bone disease. Besides, she needs to urinate frequently and is diagnosed with pneumonia and urinary tract infection. Since she doesn't have any immediate family member, she needs a bath seat and safety rails in the bathroom. What's more, she needs a nurse to visit her twice a week to monitor the medications. Finally, she needs physiotherapy 3 times a week.

By the way, she is a very independent-minded woman who is fully alert and articulate.

METS(二级)样卷(B)

Ⅰ. Listening

Part 1　1．B　2．D　3．A　4．G　5．E

Part 2　6．B　7．B　8．A　9．A　10．A

Part 3　11．A　12．A　13．C　14．B　15．A

Part 4　16．Stephen　17．30th of November, 1934　18．463817　19．morphine　20．BP/

Blood Pressure

Ⅱ. Reading and Writing

Part 1

21. C 查找：There was a tremor affecting mainly her right hand.

22. D 查找：She was sleeping poorly...

23. A 查找：She had gained 9kg in weight.

24. B 查找：...had lost about 5kg in weight.

25. A 查找：...complained of tiredness and malaise.

26. D 查找：...complaining of increased tiredness.

27. F 查找：She had had a normal pregnancy when she was 25.

28. A 查找：...her hair had started to fall out.

29. E 查找：He had noticed some swelling ankles...

30. B 查找：complaining of a painless lump on the right side of his neck.

Part 2

文章大意：本文介绍了术前评估的重要性以及应评估的内容。

31. A "实施术前评估旨在查明病人是否适合做手术。"参见第一段中"At the pre-operative assessment it is important to check that the patient is fit for surgery."

32. B "只需要对年老病人或是有健康问题的病人准备健康检查。"参见第一段中"This is especially so as many of the patients are elderly and may have other health problems"，注意其中 as 表示原因，especially so 表示"尤其如此"，说明还有其他情况，后面谈的只是典型情况。

33. C "术前评估有一种通用的模式。"文章列举了一些情况，但未有类似评论或总结。

34. B "手术通常需用 15～20 分钟。"参见第二段"...as long as the surgery will take, typically about 15～20 minutes"，指的是局部麻醉的手术一般要需 15～20 分钟。

35. C "有严重心脏或呼吸问题的病人手术前天应该做简单的血检。"不符合原文内容。原文是说全麻手术前可能需做简单的血检，见文中第三段中"If a general anaesthetic is planned, then ... and perhaps some simple blood tests ... can be organized at the pre-operative assessment."

36. B "白内障手术可以在心脏病发作后的三个月内进行。"参见第三段中"As a general rule, a cataract operation ... should not be performed within 3 months of a heart attack or stroke."

37. A "对一些病人而言,手术会带来担心和焦虑。参见最后一段中"... the worry and anxiety of the ordeal may increase blood pressure which could place an undue strain on a recently damaged heart or circulatory system."

38. C "术前评估中也可以向病人提供心理咨询。"虽然文章最后提到担心和焦虑可能对手术的影响,但未涉及心理咨询方面的话题。

39. A "病人手术前最好制定长时段的康复计划。"参见文章结尾句。

40. C "相对局部麻醉而言,我们更建议进行全身麻醉。"文章只是在第二三段提及这两种情况,但未作出孰优孰劣的评判。

Part 3

文章大意：本文介绍了什么是急救,以及急救的作用、急救措施、急救原则、如何对受害者的状况进行迅速评估等。

41. C 问哪一项不属于急救的作用,注意 C 项中 avoid 一词,文章首句中"a victim of sudden illness or injury"指既成事实。

42. B　实施急救前应该注意的事项,参见文章第二段。

43. C　实施急救时,首先应该干什么,参见第三段 The first step is to call for Professional medical help.

44. B　对受害者的评估内容,参见第三段 The victim should be checked for a medical bracelet or card that describes special medical conditions.

45. A　本文的写作目的,从文章大意可以看出主要是普及一些急救常识。

Part 4

文章大意:本文主要介绍实施肌肉注射的步骤。

一、核对医嘱。

二、从密封瓶或安瓿中抽取正确剂量的药物。

三、如药品对皮下组织刺激性过强,注射前更换注射器上的针头。

四、选择肌肉注射部位。

五、找准注射部位,协助病人调整到合适的体位。通常病人取俯卧位,脚趾向内。

六、用消毒棉签以注射点为中心由内向外环形擦拭消毒注射部位,范围为 5 厘米。

七、去除针头帽。

八、排出针筒中的空气。

九、用非优势手绷紧注射部位皮肤。

十、用拇指和食指握住注射器,以 90 度角迅速进针。

十一、用非优势手握住针筒,用优势手向上抽动活塞。如果注射器中出现血液,拔出针头,丢弃注射器,重新准备注射。如果注射器中未出现血液,握稳注射器,缓慢匀速注射药物。

十二、注射之后按摩注射部位,促进药物吸收。

十三、注射完毕处理用物,洗手,记录,观察病人。

Part 5

文章大意:本文主要介绍骨质疏松症的易发性和预防措施。

51. C　分词短语作结果状语。

52. I　be susceptible to 表示"易于……"。

53. L　by 表示以某种方式,后面接动词的-ing 形式。

54. A　amount 表示"量"。

55. E　inevitably 表示"无法避免地"。

56. J　前部分为让步状语从句,承接上文;主句涉及的是锻炼的新话题,引领下文。

57. H　intake 为"摄入"之意。

58. F　从 also 一词可以看出该句与前一句为并列关系,所以应该填的词与前一句的 obtaining 意思一致,故选 Consuming("消耗",这里指"摄入")。

59. K　注意 this 在这儿指前面一句所提"抽烟带来的危害——加速骨质疏松"。

60. B　expose/exposure 与 to 搭配,表示"暴露于……"。

Part 6

参考样文:

Mr. Martha, 36 years of age, was admitted on 23 April, 2015, and discharged on 10 May, 2015.

The past medical history revealed a long history of IDDM (insulin-dependent diabetes mellitus) and HT (hypertension). An attack of Ml (myocardial infarction, occurred to him four months ago and therefore he underwent an operation of femoral-popliteal bypass as a treatment. He regularly takes medications of insulin, half an aspirin and a multivitamin. He has a history of allergy to penicillin and codeine. Since he doesn't have any immediate family member, he lives a quite independent life. This time, he was admitted to hospital in order to get an overall review of a venous ulcer.

课文译文

Unit 1

Part I Text

护理程序

什么是护理程序？在护理中，护理程序是护理实践的基础之一。为护士解决护理问题提供了思维框架，也有助于提高护士的批判性思维能力。需要重点指出的是，这个过程是灵活的，非僵化的。它是护理过程中使用的一种工具。

护理程序是护士为保证病人护理质量而采用的一种科学方法。缩写 ADPIE 可以帮助你记住护理程序的五个步骤，ADPIE 五个字母分别代表评估、诊断、计划、实施和评价。

评估

第一步是评估。在这一阶段，护士的工作是收集病人、家庭或护士所负责社区的数据。客观数据或通过体检收集来的数据是可以测量的，包括检查生命体征或观察病人的行为。

主观数据是通过交流收集到病人生病时的需求、感受和想法。在这一步骤中，就能获取病人对当前情况的反应的相关信息了。

诊断

第二步是诊断。护士通过护理评估收集信息、分析信息、找出问题，并运用护理干预改善患者病情。

计划

第三步是计划。护士要考虑哪些是首优护理诊断。病人可以而且应该参与这一过程。计划先从确定病人目标开始。根据护理诊断确定护理目标，目标就是护士护理病人要实现的程度——无论是短期还是长期目标都应该确立。然后，护士要制定达到这些目标所需的步骤，并做出个性化的护理干预方案。

实施

第四步是实施，就是真正执行护理干预或护理计划。常见的护理干预包括疼痛管理、手术后并发症预防、对病人进行教育和指导以及其他护理措施。

评价

一旦实施了护理干预措施，护士就要去评估病人的健康现状有没有达到预期目标。病人的结果一般可以描述成这三种状况：病情好转了；病情稳定了；以及病情恶化，病人死亡或出院了。如果病人的情况没有改善，或者如果没有达到健康目标，护理程序又回到第一步重新开始。

所有护士必须熟悉护理程序的步骤。如果你打算成为一名护士，那么在你的新职业生涯中，每天都要做好使用这些步骤的准备。

Part II Dialogue

（护士正在从病人那里获取信息）

护士：下午好，你叫李华，对吗？

李华：对的。有什么事吗？

护士：你介意我问你一些问题吗？

李华：问吧。

护士：你的身高？

李华：159 厘米。

护士：体重呢？

李华：69 公斤。

护士：有什么不舒服吗？

李华：我腹痛。

护士：从什么时候开始的？

李华：早上的时候开始的。刚开始是胃疼。

护士：持续了多久呢？

李华：大约三小时。到了今天下午就变成右下腹部疼。

护士：还有什么别的症状吗？

李华：我还感到反胃。

护士：有没有腹泻？

李华：没有。

护士：发烧吗？

李华：我不清楚。

护士：我给你量下体温。好的，你有点低烧，请躺在床上。我会让医生来给你检查腹部，不要紧张，
　　　放松。

李华：好的。

Part Ⅲ　Scene Practice

对于护理专业的学生来说，护理程序是一个容易让人混淆的概念，较难掌握。下面通过一个例子来从头到尾给大家做一个示范。

评估

约翰因为周末感到身体不适，星期一去他的内科医生那里就诊。护士把他从候诊室叫出来量了体温、心率和血压，问了他一系列他对疾病的感受的问题。约翰说他一直感到呼吸困难并且非常疲惫。护士把这些情况都一一记录下来。护士还从约翰的病史中发现他以前有胆固醇和血压方面的问题，并在医生探视期间为他采集了血样。

诊断

护士观察约翰的症状，并注意到他的心率高于平均值并且血压升高。考虑到约翰胆固醇水平过高时曾经出现疲劳和气短，护士判断他患有高脂血症，也就是血液中的脂肪含量过高。约翰的验血结果也证实了这个假设。护士认为他还有心脏病的危险。

计划

约翰星期二来到医生办公室接受随访。关上门之后，护士向约翰说明了他的胆固醇水平和高血压的情况。她建议约翰接受每周两次的药物治疗，以帮助降低血脂血压，还建议一周至少锻炼两次，护士还告诉约翰，他应该远离咸的食物，少吃红肉。约翰同意护士的意见，他们安排了两周后的随访。护士还提醒约翰如果他的病情有任何变化，或者他开始感觉更糟，要马上给医生打电话。

实施

约翰按照护士推荐的方法开始服药。一周后，他有一天感到特别不舒服，打电话到医生办公室。护士解释说，这种药物可能会有恶心的副作用，并建议约翰可以喝姜汁并避免吃任何使他的胃不舒服的食物。约翰继续服药，在两周内去了四次健身房。两周过去后，他又来到医生办公室接受随访。

评价

约翰回来后，护士问了他一些对于疾病的感受的问题。约翰回答说，自从锻炼和服用药物了之后，他的呼吸更轻松了，也没有那么累了。护士在他的官方医疗记录上标出"病人的病情好转"，并祝贺约翰恢复健康。然后，她建议他继续服药一个月，并坚持锻炼。

尽管她是按照护理程序中既定步骤来完成她的护理工作的,但是她的那一套护理措施让人觉得很亲近与温暖,她护理病人很细心,很人性化。正如你所看到的,护理程序若在现实生活中多实践,感觉就像人的第二天性一样习惯成自然。

Unit 2
Part Ⅰ　Text

入院

病人的病情不同,入院方式也不同。有的病人是因为意外事故或突发疾病而入院,他们病情严重,需要紧急处理和治疗。该入院方式为急症入院。有些病人入院,并非急症,该入院方式为常规入院。

不管您是因为急症入院还是常规入院,为了能让您愉快地度过住院这段时间,我想占用您几分钟,给您简单介绍一些您在住院期间需要了解的相关内容。

1. 病房环境

每间病房都配备有以下设备:病床、呼叫系统、浴室、电视、空调、储物柜、床头柜和暖水瓶。

2. 时间安排表

请遵守我们提供的以下时间安排表的相关规定。

时 间	日 程
早上 7：00	如果护士通知说要抽血,请保持空腹。7：00 之前用已提供的容器收集自己的尿、粪便样本。
早上 8：30	医生早上 8：30 开始查房,请在这之前吃完早餐在病房等待。
中午 12：00	午餐
下午 3：00—晚上 7：30	探视时间
晚上 6：00	晚餐
晚上 9：30—10：00	睡觉(请关掉灯和电视以保持安静)

3. 预防感染

让我们携起手来共创健康环境,避免感染。

医院保洁人员每天会打扫卫生,然而,如果我们共同努力,会让我们的环境更加美好。

a）每天按时洗手。确保使用正确的肥皂洗手方式。

b）禁止抽烟。抽烟在我们医院是被严厉禁止的,因为抽烟不仅影响到您自己的身体健康,还会影响到您身边的人。

c）当您咳嗽或打喷嚏的时候,请用手捂住您的鼻子和嘴巴,以免病菌传播。

d）当您感冒或是发高烧的时,请通知我们的医护工作人员。

e）为了保护环境,请不要随地吐痰。

4. 病人的义务

为了给您提供一个和谐健康的就医环境,请配合我们做好以下几点:

a）在病房请不要高声喧哗,在您看电视或用电脑时,请把音量调到最小声。

b）住院期间请不要抽烟和喝酒。

c）请节约用水用电。

d）请保持病房干净整齐。

e）住院期间请妥善保管您的私人物品。

f）请正确使用医院提供的各种设备,不得故意损坏,如有损坏请照价赔偿。

5. 用餐

我们医院有中餐、西餐和清真食品。另外,有临床营养师指导特殊饮食。如果您不愿意在医院就餐,请联系我们的病人服务中心帮您在外面订购。

6. 外出

病人住院期间,如要离开医院,须征得主管医生的同意。

7. 病人的权利

病人有权对我们的工作提出意见或建议,请您及时把意见或建议反馈给我们的病人服务中心,便于我们能尽快采纳或改进。

Part II　Dialogue

护士:您好,格林夫人。欢迎入住我们医院,我是您住院期间的主管护士,您可以叫我玛丽。希望您住在这能有家的感觉。

病人:给您添麻烦了。

护士:别客气,这是我的工作。我带您去病房,请跟我来。这边请,这就是您的病床。

病人:请问,能告诉我如何使用控制板上的按铃吗?

护士:当然。床头的控制板上安装有呼叫系统,您有任何需要,就请按铃,护士会马上过来。

病人:好的。可以让我丈夫过来陪我吗?

护士:可以,但是床位费自理,但我们认为没有必要,您的情况并没有那么严重。

病人:请问病人一天的时间安排是怎样的?

护士:病人通常是6点30分起床。早餐是7点到8点,午餐12点,晚餐6点。医生8点30分开始查房。午饭过后您可以休息一会,下午3点到7点30分是探视时间。9:30—10:00为睡觉时间。

病人:不错,很合理的时间安排。

护士:为了便于护理,我需要就您的健康状况问您几个问题,可以吗?

病人:当然可以。

护士:谢谢。首先,我要查一下您的体温、呼吸、心率和血压等。请把体温计放在腋下。好了,低烧,其他一切正常。今天是因为什么来住院?

病人:我想我可能是患了流感。

护士:那你有什么症状?

病人:我全身发冷,头疼得厉害,喉咙也痛。

护士:那您之前去看过医生吗?

病人:去了,他给我开了一些药,但我感觉没有什么作用。

护士:您之前患过心脏病、糖尿病、高血压、肺炎、哮喘、肾炎、精神病等疾病吗?

病人:没有。

护士:您曾经做过手术吗?

病人:没有。

护士:您对什么药物或食物过敏吗?

病人:没有。

护士:接下来,我想了解您的家族史。您的父母是否健在?

病人:都去世了。

护士:什么原因?

病人:我母亲死于车祸,我父亲死于高血压。

护士:您还有什么其他不舒服的吗?

病人:我的鼻子塞得厉害。

护士:好的,我现在就去通知医生。这有一瓶水,您必须大量喝水,每天至少2 000毫升。您还应该清淡饮食。始终保持您的皮肤和衣服干燥。

病人：没问题。

护士：对了,明天早上抽血之前请不要再吃任何东西。我们将通过验血提供一些对症治疗的有用信息。

病人：好的。

护士：放松心情,祝您早日康复。如您有任何需要,请按铃。再见。

病人：再见。

Part Ⅲ　Scene Practice

入院流程

1. 病人持住院证到病房,护士站起,微笑,热情迎接病人,让病人坐下,给病人提供热水一杯。

2. 责任护士 5 分钟内准备好床铺,送病人到病床,做入院介绍(管床医生及护士、病区环境、订餐及打开水时间、安全制度、贵重物品保管、传呼器的应用等)。

3. 责任护士填写住院病历、住院一览牌及床头卡。

4. 完成护理体检(体温、脉搏、呼吸、血压、体重等)。

5. 通知医生查看病人。待医嘱出来后,立即给病人做治疗。

6. 责任护士 4 小时内完成首次护理记录,8 小时内与病人进行有效的交流与沟通,了解其个性心理、生理状态与需求,实施针对性的护理。

7. 护士长对白天入院的病人 8 小时内,晚间入院的病人 14 小时内,到病人床前问候并做自我介绍。

8. 急诊送入病房抢救的病人,不需通过住院登记办理住院手续,由绿色通道人员及急诊科医护人员直接护送进入病房,其入院手续由家属或工作人员到住院处补办。

9. 严格执行病人入院"八个一"服务：

　　一个热情的问候;

　　一个亲切的称呼;

　　一张真诚的笑脸;

　　一张整洁的病床;

　　一杯温热的开水;

　　一次耐心周到的入院介绍;

　　一次准确规范的入院评估;

　　一次详细全面的健康宣教。

Unit 3

Part Ⅰ　Text

生命体征

生命体征包括体温、呼吸频率、脉率和血压。这些数据提供了病人健康状况的重要信息(也因此称为"至关重要"),尤其能识别出存在的急性疾病。

生命体征指标越危险,病人的病情越严重。

许多因素可引起生命体征改变,例如,睡眠、饮食、天气、噪音、运动、药物、恐惧、焦虑和疾病,有时会超出正常范围。

1. 体温

体温通常用带电子读数的口腔温度计,放在舌下来测量。这样测量到的是口腔温。其他两个常用来测量体温的部位有直肠和腋窝。

温度的测量标准有两种：华氏和摄氏。成人正常的平均口腔温为 98.6℉(37℃);肛温为 99.6℉(37.5℃);腋温为 98℉(36.7℃)。

许多因素,如年龄、感染、环境温度、运动量、精神状态会影响病人的体温,因此测评体温时要考虑到这些因素。例如,体温最低时出现在早上2点至6点;最高时在下午4点至8点。

选择合适的方法来测量体温取决于几个因素,如病人的年龄、意识水平和精神状态。口腔温测量不适用于儿童,意识错乱及或无意识的病人,或者口腔疼痛、创伤或发炎的病人。

2. 呼吸频率

呼吸是指把空气中的氧气吸入肺部并把二氧化碳排出肺部的过程。当吸气时,胸腔扩张。当呼气时,胸腔收缩。

呼吸频率按每分钟呼吸的次数来记录。成人休息时的正常呼吸频率为每分钟呼吸16～20次。当你在数呼吸次数时,尽量小心翼翼以避免病人知道别人正在测量其呼吸。正确方法是在你测完脉搏后仍然把手放在病人的手腕上,数病人的胸部起伏次数30秒,然后乘以2,再做记录。在测量期间,需要用到秒表。

呼吸特征的描述可以采用不同的术语。例如,dyspnea用来描述呼吸困难,apnea指缺乏呼吸,tachypnea则指呼吸过快。

3. 脉率

脉率是指心率,或指一分钟内心跳的次数。脉搏跳动的强弱和节奏也必须要观察和描述。正常脉率跳动均匀规则,间隔时间相等。正常脉率是每分钟60～100次。

只要有大动脉的部位(如颈动脉、股动脉,或者只需听心跳)都可以测量脉率,但为方便起见通常取腕动脉来测量。首先轻轻按压,当皮下脂肪厚或感觉不到脉搏的时候用点力按压。如果按压腕动脉过度,会使血管闭塞而导致测出的脉率不准。

4. 血压

血压是心脏喷射的血液在动脉血管壁上所呈现出来的压力。

测量血压有两个数值,较高的称为舒张压,较低的称为收缩压。正常的血压范围从110到140毫米汞柱(心脏收缩时)和60到90毫米汞柱(心脏舒张时)。血压通常写作120/80 mmHg,正常为100/60和140/90。收缩压高于140或舒张压高于90都属于高血压。收缩压低于100叫作低血压,不需要进行治疗。

血压变化受几个因素的影响,如年龄、运动、情绪和疼痛。

测量血压需要一条袖带和一个血压计。应正确使用这些工具,否则会影响读数的准确性。

Part Ⅱ　Dialogue

(一个护士正在内科病房里检查病人的生命体征)

护士:早上好。我是您的责任护士王梅。您今天感觉如何?

病人:早上好。我今天感觉好多了。

护士:太好了,我准备检查您的生命体征。

病人:好的。

护士:在过去的30分钟里您做过剧烈运动吗?吃过冷的或热的食物或水吗?有没有洗澡呢?

病人:没有。我是在40分钟前吃的早餐。

护士:好的。首先让我来测量您的体温。请把体温计放在您的腋下。

病人:体温计在腋下需放置多久?

护士:大约10分钟。现在请伸出您的手腕,我要测量您的脉搏和呼吸。

(10分钟后)

病人:我的体温、脉搏和呼吸怎么样?

护士:您的体温是36.5℃,脉率每分钟90次,呼吸每分钟20次。一切正常。

病人:好的。谢谢你。

护士:不用谢。我还要测量您的血压。请您卷起衣袖,稍许抬起手臂,以便我绑袖带。

病人:没问题。

护士:您可能会感觉手臂会有点紧,请放松。

（几秒钟后）

护士：您的血压是120/85。我来帮您放下衣袖。

病人：血压正常吗？

护士：血压处于正常范围。您的生命体征很好。好的，检查完毕。

病人：很高兴听到这消息。

护士：这是呼叫铃。如果您有任何需要，请按铃。我会马上回来。祝您愉快！

病人：好的。谢谢你，王梅。

护士：不客气。

Part Ⅲ Scene Practice

血压测量

一、目的

了解收缩压和舒张压的变化，观察病情，协助诊断与治疗。

二、准备

1. 护士准备：着装整洁，洗手，戴口罩。

2. 患者准备：体位舒适，情绪稳定，活动、进餐后需休息半小时。

3. 用物准备：台式汞柱血压计、听诊器、笔、护理记录单。

4. 环境准备：病室清洁、安静、光线适宜。

三、操作标准

实　施	护理用语
1. 备齐用物携至患者床旁。查对床号、姓名，询问患者活动情况，必要时休息片刻后再测（一般要求患者安静休息5～10分钟）。 2. 选择血压测量部位（肱动脉），测血压。 3. 协助患者取舒适坐位或卧位，卷袖充分暴露一侧上臂（一般为右上臂；偏瘫、肢体外伤或手术的患者选择健侧肢体；输液肢体一般不选用测量）。 4. 协助患者伸直肘部并稍外展，手掌向上。 5. 血压计平放，位置与肱动脉、血压计零点、心脏在同一水平线上。 6. 打开血压计，驱净袖带内空气，并将袖带平整无折地缠于上臂，松紧以放入1指为宜，使球囊的中央放在手的内侧面，其下缘成人距肘窝2～3 cm。 7. 打开汞槽开关，戴好听诊器，在肘窝部扣及肱动脉搏动，将听诊器胸件紧贴肱动脉明显处。 8. 关闭气门，缓慢打气至动脉搏动消失，再上升20～30 mmHg（2.7～4 KPa）后慢慢打开气门使汞柱缓慢下降，以每秒钟下降4 mmHg为宜。注意汞柱刻度和肱动脉声音的变化，第一声为收缩压，变声或声音消失为舒张压（测量要准确，充气不可过猛或放的速度不宜过快，当舒张压声音突然变小或消失差异很大时都应记录）。 9. 重测时，先将袖带内空气驱尽，使汞柱下降至零点，稍等片刻再进行第二次测量，连续测量2～3次，取最低值。 10. 测量结束，排尽袖带内余气，血压计盒盖右倾45度，使汞全部回流到汞槽内，关闭汞槽开关，盖上盒盖，平稳放置。 11. 整理床单位和用物。 12. 洗手，记录血压。	——您好，赵女士。我要给您测血压了。 ——您躺在沙发上，然后放松。 ——现在请您伸出手臂，掌心向上。 ——如果您觉得不舒服，请告诉我。 ——您的血压是120/80，属于正常范围。如果您需要任何帮助，请按铃。我会马上过来，好好休息。

Unit 4
Part I Text

给药途径

给药途径在药理学和毒理学中指药物、液体、毒或其他物质被施入体内的路径。给药途径一般根据物质的施用部位来分类。常见的例子包括口服和静脉给药。给药途径也可以基于给药的目标位置来分类。给药可以是皮肤的（局部的）、肠内的（全身性作用，但通过胃肠道递送）或胃肠外的（系统性作用，但通过除胃肠道其他途径递送）。

给药可以通过不同的方式实施。

A. 口服用药是最常见的方式，即通过口腔给药。任何通过口腔的给药都可以看作是口服药。即便药物的吸收始于口腔，但大部分在胃或肠中吸收。它可分为：

1. 舌下用药：药物放在舌头下面，药物被吸收到舌头下面血管里。

2. 口腔用药：对颊黏膜口内进行用药。含片往往是硬片(4 小时的溶解时间)，旨在慢慢溶解。

口服用药的优势：

● 首过——对颊黏膜给药，可以避开肝脏的首过效应，因而没有药物的损失。

● 快速吸收——因为良好的血液供应，该区域的药物吸收通常相当迅速。

● 药物稳定性——pH 值在口腔相对呈中性(见胃—酸性)。因此，药物更稳定。

B. 鼻胃管给药：

   1. 指征

      1) 胃正常排空

      2) 胃没有原发疾病

   2. 优点

      1) 容易插管

      2) 完整的咽反射

      3) 无食管反流

      4) 胃有较大的容量

C. 局部给药：药剂施用到皮肤和黏膜组织上吸收，或用于局部治疗。除了施用到皮肤上，局部用药还包括：

   1. 眼部用药(药物施用到眼睛里)；

   2. 耳部用药(药物施用到耳朵里)；

   3. 鼻部用药(药物放入到鼻子里)(见图 1)；

   4. 阴道用药(药物放入阴道里)；

   5. 直肠用药(药物插入或灌入直肠里)；

   6. 肺部用药(药物吸入到呼吸道里)。

D. 胃肠外给药：即通过针头注射给药。胃肠外用药是吸收最快的，因为它们直接进入或是接近血液循环。胃肠外给药途径包括：

   1. 皮下注射(SC)途径：通过皮下组织，在皮肤下给药；

   2. 静脉注射(IV)途径：通过静脉给药；

   3. 肌肉注射(IM)途径：通过肌肉给药(见图 2)；

   4. 皮内注射(ID)途径：通过表皮，进入真皮给药；

   5. 动脉注射(IA)途径：通过动脉给药；

   6. 心内注射途径：通过心脏肌肉给药；

   7. 骨内注射途径：通过骨头给药；

   8. 鞘内注射途径：通过椎管给药；

   9. 硬膜外注射途径：椎管内硬膜外间隙的给药(见图 3)。

Part Ⅱ Dialogue

静脉输液

护士：上午好，你是38床的张女士吗？该给你做静脉输液了。

病人：什么是静脉输液？

护士：就是通过一个很小的针头，将瓶子中的液体直接滴入你的静脉内。

病人：瓶子里面是什么？

护士：是葡萄糖。手术后你还不能直接进食，所以就由它来给你提供营养。

病人：疼吗？

护士：别担心，不用紧张。针头刚进入时，会有点不舒服，但是只要扎进去了，就不疼了。

（护士在她的左臂扎上止血带，在其左手上寻找合适的静脉）

护士：请把手握成拳头状，我已经找到了进针点，让我先用碘和酒精在这消毒。好的，你会感到针刺的感觉，我让你动之前，请别动。针已经扎进去了。现在我来打开调节器，请先别动，我要把它固定好。好了，你现在可以移动了。记住保持手臂的位置低于心脏，输液的速度只能这么快了，自己不要随意调节滴速。

病人：为什么不让药液滴得快些呢？

护士：静脉输液必须滴得慢一些，不然的话会加重心肺的负担。如你觉得这儿疼痛，有灼热感或红肿，请立刻叫我们。我们会定期过来查看血液是否回流，药液是否滴完。

Part Ⅲ Scene Practice

青霉素过敏皮试

目的：测试身体对青霉素的过敏。

准备：

1. 护士：穿上护士服，带上护士帽，穿上鞋子和戴上口罩。修整指甲和洗手。

2. 病人：给病人解释皮内注射的目的和实施准则。

3. 设备：1毫升无菌注射器，5毫升无菌注射器，无菌容器和无菌镊子，消毒棉签，75%酒精，碘伏，青霉素（800 000 U），托盘，消毒纱布，无菌生理盐水，砂带，无菌包装盒，急救箱，包括2支肾上腺素，1支地塞米松，砂带，无菌纱布，2支无菌注射器（2—5毫升），开瓶器。

4. 环境：环境应该干净、宽敞和明亮。

标准和步骤：

实　　施	护理用语
（1）检查医嘱，使用无菌处理托盘。 （2）皮试液的配置： 　①检查药物，常规消毒青霉素药瓶及生理盐水安瓿，并折断安瓿。 　②检查注射器，用5 ml注射器抽吸等渗盐水4 ml注入青霉素瓶中，充分溶解。 　③用1 ml注射器抽吸青霉素液0.1 ml，另抽等渗盐水0.9 ml摇匀；再推掉青霉素液，剩0.1 ml，再抽等渗盐水0.9 ml摇匀；再推掉青霉素液，剩下0.1 ml/0.25 ml，再抽等渗盐水0.9 ml/0.75 ml摇匀（配置成200 U/ml或500 U/ml）。 　④更换新针头；用塑料盖盖上，防止污染针头，然后把它放在一个无菌处理托盘上。 （3）安排一套设备，按顺序放在一个托盘上，把它带到病人的床边，给病人讲解注射的目。读取病人的床卡后，重新检查病人的病史、过敏史及家族史。	——刘丽，你好，吃过早餐了吗？现在我想给你做一个皮试。 ——请放松，不要紧张。让我帮你卷起袖子。

（续表）

(4) 协助病人采取舒适的姿势,挽起袖子至肘部,选择注射部位(前臂内侧骨下三分之一),用75%酒精清洁注射部位(避免使用碘消毒液,酒精过敏者用生理盐水擦拭清洁皮肤),排出气泡,并重新检查。 (5) 左手绷紧前臂掌侧皮肤,右手持注射器,针头斜面向上与皮肤呈0—5度角刺入,至针头斜面完全进入皮内。左手拇指固定针栓,右手推入药液0.1 ml,使局部变成一圆形隆起的皮丘,且皮丘皮肤变白,毛孔变大。 (6) 快速拔出针头。 (7) 告知病人注意事项。 (8) 再次检查,拿走设备,整理床位。 (9) 20分钟后,观察结果(阴性反应:圆形小包没有变化;圆形小包的周围组织没有发红、伪足和发痒,患者没有任何不舒服的感觉;阳性反应:圆形小包的直径超出1 cm,圆形小包周围的组织发红,有伪足和瘙痒;病人感觉闷热,头晕;甚至发生过敏性休克)。 (10) 记录(阴性为"－"和阳性为"＋"),若为阳性,给病人和家属一个明确的解释,并在输液卡、医嘱、显示板、床头卡和医疗卡上记录清楚。	——你有什么不舒服吗? 20分钟后我会来看结果,同时请不要离开病房,不要按或是抓皮试的地方。如有不适,请尽快告诉我们。 ——刘丽,你感觉好吗? 有什么不舒服吗? 让我看一下结果,你的皮试结果是阴性的,我们将给你注射盘尼西林。

Unit 5
Part Ⅰ　Text

肠道喂养

无论患什么病,病人都需要充足的营养去恢复健康。重病患者对营养的需求更高并容易在短时间内产生营养不良的情况。研究表明,早期喂养对病人的康复很重要。所有病人的营养需求情况每天都要检查,通常入院的第一天就尽快给病人提供营养治疗。肠道喂养指的是将病人所需的所有营养物质,如蛋白质、碳水化合物、脂肪、水、矿物质和维他命,直接输送至胃部、十二指肠或空肠。

喂养病人的最好方法就是利用他们自身的胃肠系统。利用胃肠系统进行喂养称之为肠道喂养,也就是通过肠子提供营养。如果当病人喉咙插入了吸气管而不能吞咽食物,就只能通过饲管进行喂养。针对这种情况设计的解决方法给病人提供了康复所需的营养物质。

胃肠管喂养对不愿自主进食者,患有长期的神经性或机械性吞咽困难,肠功能障碍以及重症患者的治疗具有非常重要的作用。大部分喂养管是从鼻子或嘴巴插入然后伸入到胃中。喂养物混合起来装入无菌袋,每天24小时给病人匀速输入。用一个类似静脉输液泵的装置进行喂养物的输送。

Part Ⅱ　Dialogue

医生:有什么不舒服吗?
病人:我最近消化不良。
医生:消化系统怎么不好受?
病人:吃进的东西都停在这里(指胸部)。
医生:什么时候觉得难受
病人:饭后两三个小时。
医生:怎么不好? 疼痛吗?
病人:是的,很痛。
医生:怎么个痛法? 烧痛还是刺痛?
病人:肠胃里胀气,我想把气排掉。
医生:打嗝吗?

病人：不常打嗝。

医生：夜间犯病吗？

病人：不。

医生：饥饿时发作吗？

病人：对，饥饿时胃部特别疼痛，如果不马上吃些东西，我就支持不住。

医生：胃口怎么样？

病人：很差。

医生：胃口一向不好吗？

病人：不，10年前才开始疼的。

医生：近几个月变化大吗？

病人：服药后，食物能够往下走了，我也感觉到饿了。

医生：你最好做一下检查，检查后我再给你开些药。

病人：需要注意些什么吗？

医生：不要吃生冷和刺激性食物。

Part Ⅲ　Scene Practice

目的：掌握鼻胃管插管操作步骤

准备：

1. 护士：收集所有所需器械并放置在一个干净的托盘中，将手完全洗净，干燥后戴上无菌手套和口罩。

2. 器械：大小及型号合适的管子、无菌水、箔碗、纱布、pH试纸、20 ml的注射器、无菌手套、胶布。

3. 环境：一间整洁安静的病房。

标准及步骤：

1. 根据患者的年龄和配合度找到最佳的插入位置。确定选择插入的鼻孔干净无污物，如果年龄允许，询问病人愿意将鼻管插入哪边。

2. a. 检查管子是否完整无损。将管子伸展开而不要保持包装时的形状，如果管子有导丝，要确认好导丝是否正确插入管子而没有弯曲。如果管子含有导丝，在插入前用 10 ml 的无菌水冲洗管子。

　　b. 给婴儿或小孩插管：测量需要插入的管子长度。先测量从鼻骨至耳垂的长度，再测量从耳垂至剑胸骨长度。管子的长度可以使用不掉色的笔或用胶布在管子上做记号。

　　c. 为新生儿插管：测量从鼻子至耳朵，然后再测量耳朵至剑胸骨和肚脐中间的长度。

　　d. 将管子的一端用无菌水润滑，不要使用 K-Y 润滑液。

　　e. 将患者的头轻轻向前压，轻柔地将管子插入患者的鼻孔，顺着鼻咽壁向前插至口咽，这时可以让患者吞咽一些水或是给小孩安抚奶嘴，用以帮助这段管子向下插入食道直至所需长度。

　　f. 当遇到阻力的时候一定不要再向前插管。如果患者呼吸困难或剧烈咳嗽，立即将管子撤出。

　　g. 确认位置无误后，轻柔地用胶布或借助辅助物将管子固定住。

Unit 6
Part Ⅰ　Text

外科护理中护士的角色

　　卫生保健是一个庞大而复杂的体系，它既反映了社会的变化，也反映了需要健康护理的人口的变化，同时也反映了人类对身体健康的关注超过对疾病的关注。为了应对这些变化，外科护士的角色也在不断拓宽。他们是教育者、倡导者、领导者、管理者和研究者，而不再仅仅是护理者。护士们扮演这些角色来帮助人们改善健康状况，预防疾病，帮助那些需要医疗服务的成年患者来应对残疾或者死亡。

　　护士首先是护理者。尽管作为护理者所从事的活动在21世纪发生了巨大的变化，但是从1900年至

20世纪60年代以来,护士几乎都是女性,所从事的工作就是遵从医嘱从事护理工作。随着护理人员受教育程度的不断提高,护理学的不断发展以及人们逐渐认识到护士工作的自主性和专业性,他们逐步摆脱这种医生附属品的角色。

作为护理者,护士的工作具有独立性,也必须具有协助意识。护士必须根据所学的护理学知识和技能对病人做出评估,规划和实施具体的护理工作,同时还需要与医疗团队的其他成员合作,补充和评估医疗服务。

护理工作既是一门科学,也是一门艺术。在护理过程中要以批判性思维作为整个护理工作的框架,不再是单纯的疾病护理,而是以"病人及其家属"为中心的心理、文化、精神以及环境等的全方位护理,是考虑到病人各种需求的整体护理。整体护理是基于整体大于局部之和的哲学观基础之上的,同时还强调个体的独特性。

在提供全面、个性化的护理服务时,护士必须应用批判性思维去分析、综合来自于艺术和科学以及护理研究和理论的知识。在护理过程中将护理知识转化为护理艺术。护理服务是连接护理与病人的纽带,因此护士不仅要具备专业知识和技能,还应具备同情心和人文关怀的精神。

Part Ⅱ   Dialogue

(病房里,护士正在给病人做手术前的指导)

护士:李先生,你好! 正在下床活动啊(李先生点头答应),让我看看引流袋(护士弯下腰查看了尿液的引流情况)。很好,尿色也很清。你早晨喝水了吗?

病人:喝了一小杯水。护士,你能帮我给医生打个招呼,早点给我做手术吗?

护士:李先生,你不要着急,明天你就要手术了。昨天我给你介绍了手术的方法及配合手术的一些事项,你还有那些不明白的地方我再给你说说,好吗?

病人:我都明白了。你看你给我的这些资料我都反反复复看了好几遍了。我说给你听听(王先生开始复述手术的相关知识,护士边听边给予补充和纠正)。

护士:李先生,你记性真好! 那我们练习一下全身放松、深呼吸,还有咳嗽和排痰。你先躺在床上(护士扶李先生上床,李先生开始练习)。深呼吸时嘴巴闭起。对,用鼻子吸气,双手不要握拳,手掌自然伸开。好,再来一次。

护士:李先生,明天手术是硬膜外麻醉,也就是我们常说的半身麻醉。麻药打在腰脊椎骨内,下半身没有知觉,但人是清醒的。我现在教你麻醉时如何配合医生。来,把身体侧卧,双腿屈曲,靠近胸口,双手抱住膝盖。背尽量向后凸,头低下一点儿。好,就是这样。李先生,我先去看看其他病人,等一会儿我再来给你做术前准备工作,你先休息一下,与26床的张先生聊聊,他和你的手术是一样的。

(护士请26床的张先生和李先生谈手术体会,护士在做完其他病人的护理后为王先生做了常规的术前准备工作)

Part Ⅲ   Scene Practice

导尿术

目的

1. 为尿潴留患者导出尿液,以减轻痛苦。

2. 协助临床检查,如留取未受污染的尿标本作细菌培养,测量膀胱容量、压力及残余尿量,进行尿道或膀胱造影等。

3. 为膀胱肿瘤患者进行膀胱内化疗。

操作前准备

1. 护理准备:着装整洁,剪指甲,洗手,戴口罩。

2. 患者准备:让患者和家属了解导尿的目的、意义、注意事项及配合操作的要点。能下床活动的患者,嘱其自行清洗外阴;若不能,则由护士协助冲洗。

3. 用物准备:治疗盘内备无菌导尿包,内装单腔导尿管2根、血管钳2把;小药杯内放棉球数个、石蜡油棉球数个、孔巾、弯盘2个、有盖标本瓶试管、纱布数块,以及会阴消毒包;治疗碗内盛棉球数个、血管钳、纱布数块、弯盘、无菌持物钳及持物筒、一次性手套和无菌手套各一副、络合碘、弯盘、橡胶单、治疗巾、浴巾、笔、记录单、便盆及便盆巾,必要时准备屏风。按方便操作的原则放好所需用物。

4. 环境准备:关闭门窗,放下窗帘,必要时屏风遮挡,保持合适的室温。

操作标准

实施	护理用语
1. 将用物推至患者床旁,核对患者的床号和姓名,向患者解释导尿的目的。	周先生/周阿姨,您好,根据医生的医嘱要给你插导尿管,插尿管后可以帮助你把尿液引流出来。请问您清洗会阴了吗?
2. 将床尾盖被翻至患者耻骨联合上,帮助患者脱去近侧裤腿,盖在对侧腿部;近侧腿用浴巾遮盖。	我帮您脱下裤子。
3. 协助患者取屈膝仰卧,两腿略向外展,露出外阴。将橡胶单和治巾垫于患者臀下。	请你抬高臀部。
4. 清洁外阴: (1) 打开会阴消毒包,倒络合碘溶液于治疗碗内; (2) 戴一次性手套。弯盘置于外阴旁,治疗碗放在两腿之间。	
男性患者 (3) 右手持血管钳夹络合碘棉球消毒阴阜,阴茎,阴囊。左手用无菌纱布裹住并提起阴茎,将包皮向后推,露出尿道口,右手持血管钳夹络合碘棉球消毒外阴。消毒顺序:尿道口、龟头、阴茎颈、阴茎体、阴茎根部、阴囊、耻骨联合和腹股沟。每个棉球限用一次。	周先生/周阿姨,现在给您消毒外阴。
女性患者 (4) 右手持血管钳夹络合碘消毒阴和大阴唇。左手分开大阴唇,右手持血管钳夹络合碘棉球消毒小阴唇及尿道口。顺序:由外向内,自上而下。每个棉球限用一次。 (5) 用过的棉球及手套放于弯盘内,置于护理车下层。	周先生/周阿姨,现在给您消毒外阴。
5. 在患者两腿之间打开导尿包外层包步,再按无菌技术操作打开内层治疗巾,用无菌持物钳夹出小药杯至无菌巾边缘,倒络合碘溶液于小药杯内。	
6. 戴无菌手套,铺孔巾,暴露会阴,使孔巾和导尿包包布形成一个无菌区。	请您不要动,我要在两腿之间铺巾。
7. 消毒会阴及导尿插管: (1) 按操作顺序排列无菌用物,检查导管是否通畅。用石蜡油棉球润滑导尿管前段后置于弯盘内备用,将另一弯盘移至外阴处。	
男性患者 (2) 左手用无菌纱布包裹阴茎,将包皮向后推,露出尿道口。再次自尿道口向外旋转消毒。顺序:尿道口、龟头、阴茎颈、尿道口。每个棉球限用一次。	请您放松,我再给您消毒一次。
(3) 左手用无菌纱布提起阴茎与腹壁呈60°角,用血管钳夹持导尿管,插入尿道口20～22 cm,见尿液流出,再插入1～2 cm。如果插管过程中有阻力,嘱患者深呼吸,再缓慢插入,忌用蛮力。如果阻力仍然存在,应停止操作,报告责任护士。	现在给您插导尿管,请您做深呼吸。

（续表）

女性患者	请您放松,我再给您消毒一次。
(2) 用左手拇指、示指分开并固定大阴唇,右手持血管钳夹络合碘棉球分别消毒阴道口及双侧小阴唇。顺序:由上而下,由内而外。每个棉球限用一次。	
(3) 用血管钳夹持导尿管,插入尿道口 4～6 cm,见尿液流出,再插入 1～2 cm。如果插管过程中有阻力,嘱患者深呼吸,再缓慢插入,忌用蛮力。如果阻力仍然存在,应停止操作,报告责任护士。	现在给您插导尿管,请您做深呼吸。
(4) 用过的血管钳、棉球放于弯盘内,移至床尾端包布边缘处,左手固定不动。	
8. 将尿液引入无菌弯盘内。若需作尿培养,用无菌标本瓶接去中尿 5 ml。弯盘内尿液需倾倒时,夹紧导尿管,将尿液倒入便盆内,再打开导尿管继续放尿。每次放尿量不超过 1 000 ml。	周先生/周阿姨,我已经帮您导出尿液。现在帮您拔管。
9. 导尿完毕,轻轻拔出导尿管,用无菌纱布擦净外阴,撤下孔巾。	
10. 脱手套。撤去橡胶单和治疗巾。协助患者穿好裤子,处于舒适体位。整理床单位,清理用物。	谢谢您的配合,我帮您穿好裤子,请您好好休息。
11. 记录。将尿标本贴签后送检	

要求

1. 与患者有效沟通,使患者能力理解导尿的目的和注意事项,并积极配合。
2. 患者无痛苦和尿道损伤。
3. 衣、被清洁、干燥。
4. 护士操作熟练、正确、无菌观念强。
5. 注意事项:
   (1) 用物必须严格消毒灭菌,按无菌操作进行,防止尿路感染。
   (2) 保护患者隐私,耐心解释,操作环境要遮挡。
   (3) 选择光滑面粗细适宜的导尿管。插管动作轻柔,以免损伤尿道粘膜。

Unit 7
Part I   Text
产褥期妇女的护理

产褥期的护理应考虑到产妇及家庭成员的生理、心理需要,护理人员必须在准确评估产妇生理功能的基础上,提供及时、准确的护理,并根据产妇的知识水平、夫妻关系进行健康知识宣教,满足产妇情感上的需要,使新生儿健康成长。所以,产褥期护理的目的是帮助产妇及家庭成员适应新生命降临以后的父母角色转换。

1. 观察子宫复旧

在分娩 24 小时以内应及时评估子宫底的高度及观察恶露的状况。24 小时后,如果子宫收缩好,观察次数可以减少。另外应让产妇了解有关子宫复旧的知识,如恶露的观察、扪及子宫底的方法。这些知识将帮助产妇识别恶露时间延长、子宫收缩不良等异常征象,以便产妇将这些异常征象及时汇报给医护人员。

2. 会阴护理

会阴护理的方法是用温开水或低浓度的消毒液清洗外阴,清洗应从前到后,避免将水冲入阴道。教会产妇更换卫生垫前要洗手,未用的卫生巾应放在干净的袋子里,会阴垫应直接从前面向后面取下,预防对外阴、阴道的污染。

3. 乳房护理

在喂奶以前应将乳头洗净,但应避免使用肥皂,因为它会将乳头上蒙氏腺体分泌的润滑剂洗掉;喂奶以后保持乳头干燥,预防组织破损。另外,应穿戴适合乳房大小的、纯棉质的胸罩支撑胀大的乳房。

4. 一般护理

(1)营养。产褥期饮食要营养均衡、热能充足以供应母乳喂养妇女的需要。产后妇女食欲很好(尤其是母乳喂养者),在三餐间常感到饥饿。因此,应给以加餐,以保证产妇的需要。同时,产妇应多吃汤类饮食,保证充足的水分,以有利于乳汁的分泌。

(2)休息与睡眠。产褥期妇女需要足够的休息,应鼓励产妇尽可能地放松并保持良好的睡眠。在病房里,护理人员对产妇的护理应集中进行,可安排在进餐前后,探视时间。如果多个产妇共用房间,应将她们的护理集中在同一时间进行,减少对产妇睡眠的打扰。另外,应保持环境安静、舒适以促进产妇睡眠。

(3)产后早期活动与保健操。向产妇讲解产后早期活动的意义非常重要。产妇的活动量应根据产妇的情况逐渐增加。早期活动可以促进母体血液循环,减少静脉血栓的发生,有利于膀胱及胃肠道功能的恢复,减少尿潴留、腹部胀气及便秘等的发生。

产妇都应掌握产褥期保健操,它可以增强泌尿生殖膈肌肉的张力,预防产后肌肉松弛。产妇应根据身体状况,循序渐进地进行锻炼,一般从产后第2天开始,每1~2天增加1节,每节做8~16次。

(4)个人卫生。沐浴可减轻疲劳,保持清洁。没有并发症的妇女,可以在产后几小时后就进行沐浴。产后妇女第一次沐浴时,护理人员应从旁保护,同时还要提供沐浴和乳房护理方面的知识。

向产妇及家庭成员强调在接触乳房前、抱新生儿之前、换尿布和排便以后等应先洗手的重要性,并教会其洗手的方法。

(5)保持大便通畅。充足的水分及食用纤维素是预防便秘的有效措施,带皮的蔬菜、水果提供了足够的粗纤维,谷类食物中也含有丰富的纤维素;增加活动也可以促进大便的排泄,散步是最好的活动方式,散步的距离和强度以逐渐增加为宜;每天至少喝8杯水,有利于正常的大便排泄;养成规律的排便习惯也是预防便秘的方法,早餐后胃肠反射增强,此时排便较好;坐浴、冷敷均可减轻外阴伤口的疼痛,有利于大便的排出;如发生便秘,可以使用润滑剂帮助大便排出。

Part Ⅱ Dialogue

(张玲和她的实习老师江护士长正在给李太太做检查,李太太是一名初产妇,出现产前阵痛。一小时后)

江护士长:李太太,该进分娩室了。张玲,帮帮她。

张玲:好。李太太,你可以靠着我,别担心。

李太太:谢谢。我觉得没劲还晕乎乎的。

张玲:很正常,坐床上吧。

江护士长:李太太,有阵痛了吧? 等一下让它过去。张开嘴,快速而短促地呼吸。过去了吧?

李太太:嗯。

江护士长:躺下,屁股移到床边,把脚放到脚蹬上。当阵痛来时,你就向下使劲,就像上厕所那样。

李太太:又疼了。

江护士长:深吸气向下使劲! 再吸气,向下使劲! 疼痛过去了吧?

李太太:是的。

江护士长:那我们等下次阵痛。

李太太:又来了。

江护士长:深呼吸,再使劲! 再使点劲! 做得不错!

张玲:我看见孩子的头了。

(生产后的第二天早晨)

江护士长:祝贺您,李太太。是个男孩,睡得好吗?

李太太:很好,谢谢!

江护士长：我想检查一下你的宫底,看看子宫恢复得怎样? 出很多血吗?

李太太：一点点。

江护士长：让我看一下护垫,你知道怎样清洗阴部吗?

李太太：不知道。

江护士长：张玲,来给李太太做一下会阴清洗。

张玲：好的,用一块干净的湿布,从前向后向肛门方向擦,绝不能反方向换。

李太太：我知道了。

江护士长：喂奶情况怎样?

李太太：孩子吮得很有劲,可我没有多少奶。

江护士长：会有的。要把孩子的舌头放在你的奶头下,用一只手把乳房托住放在他嘴里。喂奶时, 你会感到子宫有些痛,那很正常。有问题可随时找我。

李太太：谢谢!

Part Ⅲ   Scene Practice

无菌技术是指在医疗、护理操作过程中,防止一切微生物侵入人体和防止无菌物品、无菌区域被污染的技术。使用无菌技术能减少术后感染的风险,并尽量减少医护人员接触潜在的传染性微生物。

目的

1. 保持无菌物品及无菌区域不被污染。

2. 防止病原微生物侵入或传播给他人。

准备

1. 护士准备：护士着装整洁,修剪指甲,洗手,戴口罩。

2. 用物准备：治疗车上层置无菌容器及持物钳、敷料缸、棉签、消毒剂、无菌溶液、无菌巾包、无菌碗、有盖方盘或储槽内盛无菌物品、无菌手套、弯盘、开瓶器、笔和纸、抹布,另备清洁治疗盘2个。物品应放置有序,便于操作。

3. 环境准备：环境应清洁、干燥和宽敞;操作区域要清洁、宽敞、干燥。操作前半小时停止清扫地面,并用蘸有消毒的抹布擦净治疗盘和治疗台,避免不必要的人群流动,降低室内空气中的尘埃。

操作标准

实施

1. 查看无菌物品的灭菌日期和手套号码,包布有无破损、潮湿。查看指示胶带是否变色以及无菌溶液的质量,并将物品有序摆放,符合无菌操作原则。

2. 拿起无菌巾包,解开系带,绕好并置于包下;先打开无菌巾包的远侧,再打开无菌巾包的两侧,最后打开无菌巾包的近侧;查对消毒指示卡;用无菌持物钳夹取一块无菌巾放在手上,放回持物钳;捏无菌巾包外面将余物按原样折好。

3. 单巾铺盘法

(1) 手拿无菌巾,短边朝上,用一只手在靠近散边边缘2 cm处抓住无菌巾一侧,用另一只手在对侧相同处抓住无菌巾另一侧,将其轻轻抖开,双折平铺于盘上;双手捏住无菌巾上层的两角,呈扇形折叠,开口边缘向外。

(2) 打开无菌容器,取无菌持物钳,用无菌持物钳夹取无菌物品,将无菌物品放入无菌盘的无菌区内,将无菌持物钳放回无菌容器内并松开钳轴节,盖严无菌容器(取放无菌持物钳时,钳端应闭合,垂直取放,不碰及瓶口,并始终保持钳端向下)。双手捏住无菌巾上层两角的外面,使上层与下层的边缘对齐,盖住无菌物品。将无菌巾开口处向上折两次,无菌巾两边各向下折一次,记录铺盘时间,有效期为4小时。

(3) 当打开的无菌包仍有未用完的无菌物品时必须系"一"字形带,并注明开包日期和时间,有效期为24小时。

4. 双巾铺盘法

(1) 查对无菌巾包,并按单巾铺盘法打开无菌巾包。用无菌持物钳夹取一块无菌巾放在空手上,放回持物钳,然后将无菌巾包按原样折叠好。无菌巾长边朝上,双手在两角靠近散边边缘 2 cm 处抓住无菌巾两侧,轻轻打开,将无菌巾由对侧向近侧平铺于盘上,无菌面朝上。

(2) 左手拿起无菌碗包,用右手依次打开包布的三个角并抓在左手上,再将包的第四个角一起抓住,露出无菌碗,并稳妥地将它放入无菌盘内。

(3) 仔细核对无菌溶液的名称、浓度、质量和有效期。用开瓶器打开瓶盖,用双手大拇指将瓶塞边缘上推,用右手大拇指和食指将瓶塞拔出。左手拿无菌溶液瓶,手掌紧贴瓶签,先倒少许溶液冲洗瓶口,再由原处倒出适量溶液于容器内,套上瓶塞。

(4) 用左手抓住无菌容器盖的外面将其打开,右手持无菌持物钳夹取无菌纱布,盖好无菌容器,将无菌纱布放在无菌区内,放回持物钳。

(5) 用无菌持物钳夹取另一块无菌巾放在空手上,放回持物钳,双手抓住无菌巾外面两角,轻轻打开,边缘对齐,由近侧向对侧覆盖于无菌盘上,边缘剩余部分向上反折。

(6) 消毒无菌溶液瓶盖和瓶口后盖严,注明开瓶时间后放回原处,把准备好的无菌手套放在无菌盘内。已开瓶的溶液有效期为 24 小时。

(7) 拿开无菌手套,打开治疗盘上层无菌巾的小部分,露出无菌纱布。再次核对无菌手套号码,灭菌效果和日期,解开手套袋的系带,绕好置于一侧,取出滑石粉扑在手上。持手套翻折部分,同时取出两只手套。一手伸入手套内戴好,再以戴好手套的手伸入另一手套反折部分依法戴好,将手套反折部分拉平,调节手指。从无菌盘内取纱布擦净手套上的滑石粉并双手抓碗。

(8) 操作完毕,用戴好手套的手抓住另一只手套的上端外面脱下手套,使其反面朝外;用脱掉手套的手指伸入另一只手套内面脱下手套,使其反面朝外。

5. 整理用物,将用物放回原处。

Unit 8
Part Ⅰ Text
发热患儿的护理

治疗发热是为了减轻不适。对发热的患儿首先应向医生汇报发热情况,按处方给予退热剂,同时检测患儿出入液量,以防脱水。降温的方法包括药物降温和物理降温。

物理降温的步骤为:①将婴儿的皮肤暴露在空气中,如环境太热,可用电风扇或空调,但风口不要正对患儿;②可用冰袋冷敷患儿的额头、腋下,冷敷前先用布包好冰袋,也可用 30%~50% 酒精湿敷患儿额头和四肢;③可为患儿进行温水浴:用 32~34℃ 的温水,先湿敷患儿的腋下、腹股沟、额头,并擦拭患儿四肢;④继续进行上述过程,直至体温降低为止;⑤温水浴之前和之后 30 分钟应测量生命体征。

退热药物包括扑热息痛、阿司匹林和非甾体类抗炎药。扑热息痛是优选的药物。患儿应用阿司匹林可能与感染流行性感冒病毒或水痘及 Reye 综合征有关,因此阿司匹林不应该给患儿应用。用量以最初的体温水平为基础:低于 39.2℃(102.5℉),每千克体重 5 毫克;高于 39.2℃,每千克体重 10 毫克。治疗疼痛的推荐剂量是每 6~8 小时每千克体重 10 毫克,治疗疼痛和发热的最大剂量是每天每千克体重 40 毫克。退热期大约是 6~8 小时。

退热剂可每 4 小时给药一次,但 24 小时不应超过 5 次。正常情况下体温在夜间会降低,24 小时内应给药 3~4 次通常能控制大多发热。应用退热剂后 30 分钟应再测体温以评价它的效果,但不应该过多反复地测量。患儿的不舒适水平是继续治疗的最佳指标。

高热惊厥的发病率是 3%~4%,通常在 3 个月到 5 岁的孩子身上发生。对高热惊厥的患儿,应用退热剂不能预防其复发。

Part Ⅱ Dialogue
肺炎患儿护理

护士:布朗太太,今天宝宝好一点了吗?

患儿家长:没好,反而更加厉害了。

护士：咳嗽是不是感到轻松一点了？

患儿家长：是的。

护士：有的孩子肺炎初期只是阵发性干咳。但随着时间的推移，崩解的粒细胞及被杀死的细菌、病毒形成痰液，刺激支气管引起阵发性咳嗽、咳痰。就像战场上打仗，会留下许多敌人的尸体。其实痰液就是清理战场的产物，是疾病发展的自然过程。

患儿家长：她输了三四天的液，一点效果都没有。

护士：你不要太着急，我们正在积极治疗。药物发挥作用也要一段时间，再观察观察好吗？

患儿家长：都7天多了，现在就一个孩子，我们心里着急啊。

护士：我理解你的心情，但着急解决不了问题，反而影响你自身的抵抗力。你应该更加照顾好你自己。

患儿家长：那我平时要注意些什么？

护士：平时你要注意保持室内空气新鲜，经常开窗通风。宝宝咳嗽的时候，及时拍背帮助她把痰液咳出来。拍背时注意五指并拢内屈，使手掌边缘同时接触孩子的背，引起震动，借震动作用帮助痰液排出（示范拍背的方法）。

患儿家长：好的，我知道了。

护士：像你的孩子还小，不会吐痰，一般都咽到肚子里去了，所以有时你会看到大便中有黏液样的东西，那就是痰液。

患儿家长：是啊。我还以为吃坏了呢。

护士：是的，有的孩子由于痰液刺激胃肠道或者是病毒本身的作用，有时还会拉肚子呢。不过你不要太紧张，并不是每一个孩子都会拉肚子的。现在你的宝宝还有点发热，我们会4小时给她量一次体温。你如果觉得宝宝身体烫，随时叫我们来量体温，假如体温过高，医生会让她吃退热药的，但你不要自己觉得她发热了就随便给她吃药。平时多给宝宝喝点水，出汗多时要更换衣服，或在背上垫一块干的毛巾，防止着凉。我过一会儿再来看宝宝，你有事请按铃。

Part Ⅲ Scene Practice

氧气筒给氧法

目的

1. 减轻患者呼吸困难。
2. 提高呼吸系统疾病患者的睡眠质量。
3. 提高阻塞性肺疾病患者的生命质量。

准备

1. 护士准备：着装整洁，剪指甲，洗手。
2. 患者准备：让患者理解吸氧的目的和意义，主动配合操作。
3. 用物准备：治疗盘内备小药杯（内盛冷开水）、纱布、扳手、弯盘、鼻导管、玻璃接管、棉签、胶布、别针、酒精（或松节油）、输氧卡及笔；氧气筒及氧气表、橡胶管。按方便操作的原则放好所需用物。
4. 环境准备：病房内安全、无火源和易燃物品，无人吸烟。氧气筒周围严禁放置烟火和易燃品，氧气筒至少距火炉5 m、暖气片1 m。

操作标准

实　　　施	护理用语
1. 安装氧气表 　1) 检查是否挂有"满"的标志，移开保护帽。 　2) 打开氧气筒的总开关放出少量氧气，冲走气门上的灰尘。关上总开关。 　3) 接氧气表并用扳手旋紧。	

（续表）

实　施	护理用语
4）连接通气管、湿化瓶、橡胶管和玻璃接头。 5）关流量调节阀,开总开关。 6）开流量调节阀,检查氧气流出是否通畅及全套装置是否适用,关流量调节阀,备用。 2. 携用物至患者床旁,再次核对床号、姓名,为患者解释用氧的目的。 3. 清洁鼻孔,并检查鼻中隔是否有异常,鼻腔内有无异物。准备胶布。 4. 连结鼻导管。开流量调节阀,根据病情调节流量,并检查鼻导管是否通畅。 5. 比量插入长度（约自鼻尖到耳垂的 2/3 长）,轻轻将鼻导管插入鼻腔,如无呛咳,用胶布和别针固定。 6. 记录上氧的时间及流量,将输氧卡挂在醒目的地方,交代注意事项。 7. 用氧过程中密切观察缺氧改善情况,包括呼吸、面色、神志。 8. 停氧 　1）查对床号、姓名,与患者解释停氧的原因。 　2）夹取纱布,拔出鼻导管。擦净患者鼻、面部。 　3）关总开关,放余氧。 　4）分离鼻导管。 　5）关流量调节阀。 9. 擦拭胶布痕迹。整理床单位,帮助患者取舒适卧位。 10. 记录停氧时间。 11. 整理用物。分离湿化瓶、通气管、氧气管,卸下氧表装置。污物分类处置并洗手。	——李太太,你好! 今天由我为您输氧气,吸氧后您会舒服些。请您配合。 ——李太太,我帮你检查一下鼻腔。 ——现在帮你插管了。 ——布朗太太,我已经给您吸氧。 1.氧气是易燃易爆气体,请您和您的家属不要在病房吸烟。2.请您不要随意调节流量。3.翻身时防止鼻导管脱落。4.如有不适请及时呼叫我们。我也会经常来看您的,谢谢配合。 ——布朗太太,您感觉怎么样? 唇不发绀,脸色红润,呼吸也平稳了,我将为您停氧,可以吗? ——现在请您好好休息。再见!

中心管道给氧法

目的

1. 减轻患者呼吸困难。

2. 提高呼吸系统疾病患者的睡眠质量。

3. 提高阻塞性肺疾病患者的生命质量。

准备

1. 护士准备：着装整洁,剪指甲,洗手。

2. 患者准备：让患者理解吸氧的目的和意义,主动配合操作。

3. 用物准备：治疗碗内盛有通气管、小纱布；治疗盘内放氧气表,(1/3～1/2 满)、一次性鼻导管（鼻塞式）、小药杯（内盛冷开水）、弯盘、棉签、输氧卡及笔。按方便操作的原则放好所需用物。

4. 环境准备：病房内安全、无火源和易燃物品,无人吸烟。中心供氧管道周围严禁放置烟火和易燃品,中心供氧管道至少距火炉 5 m、暖气片 1 m。

操作标准

实　施	护理用语
1. 将用物带至患者床前,核对患者床号、姓名,向患者解释用氧目的。 2. 用湿棉签检查并湿润鼻腔	——Lily 你好! 今天由我为您输氧气,吸氧后您会舒服些。请您配合。 ——我帮你检查一下鼻腔。

（续表）

3. 将流量表连接在中心供氧装置上,连接通气管、湿化瓶和一次性鼻导管。	
4. 打开流量开关。根据病情调节氧流量。检查氧气管道是否畅通。	
5. 将鼻塞塞入鼻孔,将吸氧管固定于两侧耳廓上。	——Lily,我帮你把鼻塞塞好。
6. 记录上氧时间及流量,将输氧卡挂于床头。	——Lily,我已经给你上好氧了。请您和您的家属不要在病房吸烟。请您不要随意调节流量,翻身时防止鼻导管脱落,如有不适请及时呼叫我们。谢谢配合。
7. 健康教育:向患者及家属解释吸氧的目的,交代注意事项。	
8. 观察患者缺氧改善情况,包括呼吸、面色、神志等。	——Lily,您感觉怎么样?唇不发绀,脸色红润,呼吸也平稳了,根据医嘱可以停氧了。
9. 停氧 1)根据医嘱和缺氧改善情况停氧。将用物带至患者床旁,核对床号、姓名。向患者解释停氧原因。 2)拔出鼻塞,关流量开关,取下一次性鼻导管、湿化瓶和流量表。 3)清洁鼻部,记录停氧时间。	
10. 整理床单位,处理用物。	——Lily,已经帮你停了氧气。谢谢你的配合。

Unit 9

Part I　Text

出院

（住院）病人在办理了必要的手续之后正式获准离开医院,即出院。一般来说,出院是住院病人的最后一道程序。护士必须给即将出院的病人制定出院计划并进行出院教育。

出院计划

在很多国家,出院计划是卫生系统的例行手段,是（医院）为保证病人在适当时间出院,并在出院后得到充分的服务而在病人出院前为其制定的个性化出院计划。这个计划考虑到病人出院后在社区的需要,旨在更好地协调好各方给病人提供的服务。它寻求缩小医院和病人出院后落脚处的距离,减少病人住院时间,最大限度地降低病人再入院的几率。制定出院计划需要病人、病人家属和医疗团队密切协作,帮助病人出院时获得所需帮助。护士要提前为病人出院做好计划,做到以下几点:

1. 让病人及其家人全力配合;

2. 让病人及其家人了解其健康状况并对出院一事做好准确沟通;

3. 对出院的日期和时间早做计划;

4. 做好让病人在入院高峰期到来之前出院的准备;

5. 出院前两天做好协调工作,查看是否一切都已准备就绪,以保证万事俱备,等着出院。

出院教育

病人出院时很少已经完全康复的,他们仍需有一段恢复期。为了让病人完全康复,护士要负责给病人和家属必要的指导,要设法让他们明白并记住以下的事项。（列出来打印给病人）

1. 复诊:告知病人安排好的复诊日期和时间。提醒病人需要的时候向医生咨询。

2. 服药:告知病人吃药的时间和方法。用药需小心谨慎,要教会病人如何准确用药,教他一定要按你说的做。

3. 饮食:简单描述食谱,告知病人忌用食物和每天必需的食物种类和量。

4. 减少危险因素:告知病人服药仅是治疗的一部分,减少其他危险因素也同样重要,例如:减肥（如果超重）,戒烟,避免精神压力等等。

5. 警惕不良症状:这些不良症状因人而异,包括如胰岛素等药物过敏,血染衣物或睡眠时间过长。

6. 卧床病人护理指导:指导卧床病人家属如何给病人洗澡、翻身和递便盆等。

7. 休息和活动：告知病人每天必要的休息时间和活动量。

8. 出院计划和出院指导对病人出院后的护理是非常有用的。

9. 一旦病人出了院,护士就要把病房打扫干净并铺好床铺接收新来的病人。

Part Ⅱ　Dialogue

出院教育

(李梅的指导老师谢护士正在病房示范如何对病人进行出院指导)

护士：早上好,赵女士! 今天感觉怎么样?

病人：早上好,护士! 今天感觉很不错。

护士：很好,你明天就可以出院了吧?

病人：太好了。我早就想出院了。

护士：赵女士,你出院后还需要坚持低盐饮食。

病人：为什么?

护士：你的血压仍然很高,而太多的盐会使得病情更糟糕,所以你要对食盐或含钠的食物特别小心。

病人：那我就不在食物中放盐了。

护士：很好,很多食物都含盐,这是一份清单,上面所列食物是你不宜吃的。

病人：我原来不知道大蒜也含盐。

护士：是的,大蒜也含盐。你在食用食物前需要先看看标签。这是一份新药说明,它是利尿剂,会使得你的小便增多,从而使你的血压得到控制。同时,这种药会使你丢失一定量的钾,所以你需要吃一些含钾的食物。

病人：比方说香蕉和橘子?

护士：是的,这是一份含钾的食物清单。另外,这里还有一份服药说明,要注意的是,如果某次药忘记服了,千万不要将两次药一起服。如果有什么不良征兆,请给医生打电话。

病人：如果我忘了服药,该怎么办?

护士：这里说的是不要将两次药一起服,如果是早上八点的忘记服了,就改在下午两点服药,间隔适当的时间之后再服用下午的药。你下午服药时间是几点?

病人：4：30,也就是说我那天只能服一次药了。

病人：是的,请仔细阅读这些说明,如有什么问题,可以随时问我。

Part Ⅲ　Scene Practice

把病人从轮椅转移到车上

目的：将出院时不能自行走动的病人送上车

准备工作

护士：穿上护士服和护士鞋,戴上护士帽和口罩,洗干净手;向病人解释坐轮椅去车上的程序和注意事项,让其做好准备。

病人：了解坐轮椅的行为动作,清楚坐轮椅去车上的程序和注意事项,做好准备并积极配合转移。

器械：轮椅和纸笔

环境：无障碍环境

操作标准和程序

动作

1. 打开车门

2. 把轮椅推到车门口

3. 调整轮椅高度

4. 缓缓向后推放好轮椅,以便把病人从车门放到车上(这时要注意保护好病人的头部,不让它碰到车门)。

5. 把病人从轮椅扶起来(当一个护士搀扶病人的时候,另一个护士取下轮椅的带状扣件并挪放好轮椅)。

   6. 让病人低头弓身坐到车上。

   7. 帮病人把双腿在车子里摆放好,朝前坐好。

   8. 关好车门。

   9. 如果可以,把轮椅折叠好放在车厢里。

录音文字

METS(二级)样卷(A)

This is METS - 2 Listening Test.

There are four parts in this test: Part One, Two, Three, and Four.

You will hear each part twice.

We will now stop for a moment before we start the test.

Please ask any questions now because you must not speak during the test.

Pause (10 seconds)

Now, look at the instructions for Part One.

You will hear five patients describing their pain to the nurse.

What pain does each patient have?

For questions 1 - 5, mark the correct letter A-H on your answer sheet.

You will hear each conversation twice.

Here is an example:

Nurse (Woman): Are you feeling better today, Mr. Heath?

  Patient (Man): Not really. My hands ache a lot.

Nurse (Woman): Would you like some painkillers?

  Patient (Man): Yes, please. My hands ache more in the mornings.

Pause (5 seconds)

The answer is Pain in the hands, so mark the letter F in the box.

Now we are ready to start.

Pause (5 seconds)

Conversation 1

Nurse (Woman): Are you all right, Mr. Hales?

  Patient (Man): No. I've got a really bad stomachache.

Nurse (Woman): Sit down on the bed and I'll get you some painkillers.

  Patient (Man): Thanks.

Nurse (Woman): When did you last have some tablets?

  Patient (Man): I'm not sure. I think it was a few hours ago.

Pause (5 seconds)

Repeat

Pause (5 seconds)

Conversation 2

Nurse (Woman): How are you feeling, Mr. Lan?

  Patient (Man): Not very well. Can I have some painkillers, please?

Nurse (Woman): Sure. Where does it hurt?

  Patient (Man): My lower back's really aching.

Nurse (Woman): OK, I'll get the tablets and a heat pack, too.

Pause (5 seconds)

Repeat

Pause (5 seconds)

Conversation 3

Nurse (Woman): Hello, Jack. How do you feel today?

  Patient (Man): Well. I've got a bit of a sore throat.

Nurse (Woman): I'll get you some painkiller for that.

  Patient (Man): Thanks. It's really painful. Can I have a cold drink too. Please?

Nurse (Woman): Sure. I'll get some iced water for you.

Pause (5 seconds)

Repeat

Pause (5 seconds)

Conversation 4

Nurse (Woman): So, what brings you here today, Mr. Swift?

  Patient (Man): Um. I've been having these really bad headaches.

Nurse (Woman): Go on...

  Patient (Man): Well, I keep getting them.

Nurse (Woman): Ah-huh? Can you describe them?

  Patient (Man): Um. it's quite a dull pain, but there's a constant throbbing pain as well—it builds up.

Nurse (Woman): Mm. Whereabouts do you get these headaches?

  Patient (Man): Here. around the front, around the forehead.

Pause (5 seconds)

Repeat

Pause (5 seconds)

Conversation 5

Nurse (Woman): Good morning, Mr. Bloomfield. What can I do for you?

  Patient (Man): I've been having some problems with my breathing.

Nurse (Woman): Mm-hmm. Can you tell me a little bit more about it?

  Patient (Man): Well, I keep getting breathless and wheezy in my chest. It all started about three weeks ago, and I've been coughing a lot with it. I thought it might be a cold coming on, but then after about another week I started finding it more and more difficult to catch my breath.

Nurse (Woman): Right, so you've had wheeziness and breathlessness for roughly three weeks.

  Patient (Man): Yes, give or take a day.

Pause（5 seconds）

Repeat

Pause（5 seconds）

This is the end of Part One.

Pause（5 seconds）

Now look at Part Two.

Pause（5 seconds）

Look at the six sentences for this part.

You will hear a conversation between Miles, the ward nurse, and Dr. Davis, about his patients IV infusion regimes.

For questions 6 - 10, decide if each sentence is correct or incorrect.

If it is correct, put a tick（√）in the box next to A for YES. If it is not correct, put a tick（√）in the box next to B for NO. Then mark the corresponding letter on your answer sheet.

You will hear the conversation twice.

Doctor（Man）：Hello, Miles. Are you looking after Mrs. Cohen today?

Nurse（Woman）：No, that's Jane, but she's just gone down to x-ray with a patient.

Doctor（Man）：Oh, I wanted to review Mrs. Cohen's IV fluids.

Nurse（Woman）：I'm looking after Jane's patients while she's away. Do you want me to pass on any updates?

Doctor（Man）：Yeah, thanks. Could you take down Mrs. Cohen's IV when is finished, please?

Nurse（Woman）：Sure. I'll just write a note about in for Jane. What about the cannula? Do you want it left in?

Doctor（Man）：I think so. Leave it for another day in case she needs some more fluids.

Nurse（Woman）：OK. Do you want to see Mrs. Smith in the next room, too?

Doctor（Man）：Yes, I need to see her. According to her blood results, her potassium levels are quite low. I'll put in a cannula when I finish my rounds. Could you start her on a litre of Normal Saline with 40 millimols of KCl?

Nurse（Woman）：OK. Here's the Prescription Chart for you to fill out.

Doctor（Man）：Thanks. That saves me a bit of leg work. Can you run it over eight hours, please?

Nurse（Woman）：Sure. One lite of Normal Saline with 40 milimols of KCl over eight hours.

Doctor（Man）：Oh. I'll have to order her some IV anibiotics. too.

Nurse（Woman）：Yeah. OK. We'll run them through a secondary line. The primary line will have the KCl running through, so we won't mix the solutions in the same line.

Doctor（Man）：Great. Now there's just Mr. Clark left. How is he?

Nurse（Woman）：He's one of Jane's patients, too. He's pretty good. He's going home today, I think.

Doctor（Man）：Yes, that's right. He's ready for discharge. Can you take out his cannula before he goes home, please?

Nurse（Woman）：Yes, sure, we can do that. I'll pass on your instructions to Jane when she gets back.

Pause（5 seconds）
Repeat
Pause（5 seconds）
This is the end of Part Two.
Pause（5 seconds）

Now look at Part Three.
You will hear a conversation between Louisa, the ward nurse, and Gina, about her operation.
*For questions 1 – 15, choose the correct answer **A**, **B** or **C**. Put a tick（√）in the box. Then mark the corresponding letter on your answer sheet.*
You will hear the conversation twice.
Pause（5 seconds）

Nurse（Woman）：Hello. Gina. I'll be looking after you today. I want to have a talk about your operation tomorrow.

Patient（Woman）：Oh. Is everything all right?

Nurse（Woman）：Yes, everything's fine. There are no problems. I just want to go through what will happen when you come back to the ward after the operation. People always feel better when they know what to expect.

Patient（Woman）：Oh, yes, you're right. I'm so nervous about the operation. I haven't been in a hospital since I was a kid, when L broke my leg. Things have probably changed a lot since then.

Nurse（Woman）：Well, hospitals have changed a bit, but don't worry. I'll go through it all now, and you'll have the opportunity to ask as many questions as you like.

Patient（Woman）：Thanks. I feel silly being so worried. I'm not normally like this.

Nurse（Woman）：That's Ok, Gina. It's quite normal to feel a bit worried. Um, I'll try and cover everything so you're prepared for what'll happen after the operation. Um, I see you've brought the leaflet about keyhole surgery.

Patient（Woman）：Yes. um, it was sent to me at home last week. The only thing I know is that I won't have a big cut so the operation won't leave a big scar.

Nurse（Woman）：That's right. Um. keyhole surgery is also called minimally invasive surgery because it's performed with the use of a laparoscope, using small incisions or surgical cuts. They are just small holes made near your navel. And you'll have a small dressing covering the holes made during the surgery. It's just a light covering to keep the area clean until it heals.

Patient（Woman）：Oh.

Nurse（Woman）：During the operation. the surgeon uses a laparoscope, which is passed through the holes to visualize your gallbladder. The infected gallbladder is removed through the largest puncture site. You'll have a mini-drain which will only stay in for a couple of hours. It's a small plastic container attached to some tubing which takes away any excess blood from your wound.

Patient（Woman）：Ah-hah. There won't be lots of blood, will there? I can't stand the sight of blood.

Nurse（Woman）：No，not much，but I can make a note for the rest of the staff to cover the drain for you so you don't see any of it.

Patient（Woman）：Thanks.

Pause（5 seconds）

Repeat

Pause（5 seconds）

This is the end of Part Three.

Pause（5 seconds）

Now look at Part Four.

You will hear a nurse getting personal details from a patient.

Listen and complete questions 16 – 20 on your answer sheet.

You will hear the conversation twice.

Nurse（Woman）：Come in，Mr. Green. Come and sit down here. So，what's your first name?

Patient（Man）：It's Peter.

Nurse（Woman）：That's P-E-T-E-R. Is that right?

Patient（Man）：Yes.

Nurse（Woman）：Well，how are you feeling，Mr. Green?

Patient（Man）：I've been having pain，pain in my chest.

Nurse（Woman）：Yes，now when did you first notice this pain?

Patient（Man）：Er，well，I suppose about six months ago.

Nurse（Woman）：And can you remember when it first came on?

Patient（Man）：Yes，well I remember. I got a bad pain in my chest when I was shopping. It was so bad that I couldn't breathe and ...

Nurse（Woman）：And where，in which part of your chest did you feel the pain?

Patient（Man）：Well，right across my chest.

Nurse（Woman）：And how long did it last?

Patient（Man）：Ooh，about ten minutes.

Nurse（Woman）：And what did you do when it happened?

Patient（Man）：I had to stop and wait for it to go away.

Nurse（Woman）：So，have you had this，the pain again since then?

Patient（Man）：Yes，I often get it when I overdo things，and when I...

Nurse（Woman）：Well，I think at this stage I'd like to examine you，your chest. So if you could strip to your waist?

Patient（Man）：Right. There we go.

Nurse（Woman）：That's fine. I'll just check your pulse first of all. Fine. That's fine. It's quite normal，70 per minute.

Patient（Man）：Er，right.

Nurse（Woman）：Now your blood pressure. Fine. That's quite normal too，130 over 80.

Patient（Man）：Oh，I'm pleased to hear it.

Nurse（Woman）：Now you're going to take deep breaths in and out while I check your lungs. In. Out. In. Out. Fine. They're completely clear. Well，Mr. Green，the pain you've been having sounds very much like the pain of what we call angina, and this, well, this occurs when not enough oxygen is getting to the heart. Now I'd like to make a few tests, and, following that I'll be able to advise some treatment for you.

Pause（5 seconds）
Repeat
Pause（5 seconds）

This is the end of Part Four.
You now have five minutes to write your answers on the answer sheet.
Pause（4 minutes）You have one more minute.
Pause（60 seconds）

This is the end of the listening test.

METS(二级)样卷(B)

This is METS-2 Listening Test.
There are four parts in this test: Part One, Two, Three, and Four.
You will hear each part twice.
We will now stop for a moment before we start the test.
Please ask any questions now because you must not speak during the test.

Pause（10 seconds）

Now, look at the instructions for Part One.

Pause（5 seconds）

You will hear five patients complaining of their sufferings to the nurse.
What does each patient complain of?
For questions 15, mark the correct letter A-H on your answer sheet.
You will hear each conversation twice.

Here is an example：

Nurse（Woman）：Are you feeling better today, Mr. Wood?
　Patient（Man）：Not really. My hands ache a lot.
Nurse（Woman）：Would you like some painkillers?
　Patient（Man）：Yes, please. My hands ache more in the mornings.

Pause（5 seconds）
The answer is Pain in the hands, so mark the letter F in the box.
Now we are ready to start.

Pause（5 seconds）

Conversation 1

Nurse（Woman）：What seems to be the problem at the moment，Mr. Hales?

Patient（Man）：Well，I've been feeling so poorly recently.

Nurse（Woman）：Feeling so poorly? What do you mean by that?

Patient（Man）：I've been getting very short of breath.

Nurse（Woman）：Hm... How long has this been going on?

Patient（Man）：For about 18 months，I think.

Pause（5 seconds）

Repeat

Pause（5 seconds）

Conversation 2

Nurse（Woman）：Do you feel any pain，Mr. Lan?

Patient（Man）：Oh，yes，quite a bit.

Nurse（Woman）：Could you show me where it hurts?

Patient（Man）：Right here，in my chest. Occasionally it moves around.

Nurse（Woman）：OK，I see.

Pause（5 seconds）

Repeat

Pause（5 seconds）

Conversation 3

Nurse（Woman）：Hello，Jack. How do you feel today?

Patient（Man）：Well，I've got a bit of headache.

Nurse（Woman）：Can you point out the painful area?

Patient（Man）：It seems to be on the right side of my head.

Nurse（Woman）：How long does the headache last when you get it?

Patient（Man）：It varies. It can be between half an hour and four or five hours.

Pause（5 seconds）

Repeat

Pause（5 seconds）

Conversation 4

Nurse（Woman）：Do you ever suffer from dizziness，Mr. Swift?

Patient（Man）：Yes，quite often.

Nurse（Woman）：When does this happen?

Patient（Man）：When I get up too quickly.

Nurse（Woman）：Do you feel as if you are falling in a certain direction?

Patient（Man）：No，not really.

Nurse（Woman）：Does the dizziness feel like spinning or is it just a kind of unsteadiness?

Patient（Man）：It feels more like spinning.

Pause（5 seconds）

Repeat

Pause（5 seconds）

Conversation5

Nurse（Woman）：Good morning. Mr. Bloomfield. Have you got any fever recently?

Patient（Man）：Yes, I've been feeling quite flushed lately.

Nurse（Woman）：Mm-hmm. Is your temperature high all the time or does it go up and down?

Patient（Man）：Well, it usually goes up at night. but it's still high even during the day...

Nurse（Woman）：What is the highest and the lowest it has been in the past few days?

Patient（Man）：The highest was 39.5℃. and the lowest was 38℃.

Pause（5 seconds）

Repeat

Pause（5 seconds）

This is the end of Part One.

Pause（5 seconds）

Now look at Part Two.

Pause（5 seconds）

Look at the six sentences for this part.

You will hear a conversation between Sophie, the ward nurse, and Mr. Jones, the patient, about wound management.

For questions 6 – 10, decide if each sentence is correct or incorrect. If it is correct. put a tick（√） in the box next to A for YES. If it is not correct, put a tick（√）in the box next to B for NO. Then mark the corresponding letter on your answer sheet.

You will hear the conversation twice

Nurse（Woman）：Hello, Mr. Jones. My name's Sophie. I'm the wound management Clinical Nurse Specialist here.

Patient（Man）：Oh. Hello, Sophie.

Nurse（Woman）：I believe you've been having a rough time with your leg wound. Would you mind if I have a quick look at it?

Patient（Man）：No, no, no. I don't mind.

Nurse（Woman）：Now. While I take This dressing off, tell me how you've been managing at home.

Patient（Man）：Oh. Well, you know. It's a bit hard on my wife. She doesn't cope with things very well. I've been doing most of the things around the house for the past few years, but I can't do much now. I've had a difficult time with this wound. I've tried my best. but I just cant do it on my own. What do you think I should do with this ulcer.

Nurse（Woman）：Well. I think the first thing to do is to eases the wound. Sometimes you have to come into hospital to get back on track with treatment. Ok, I think that we need to use a different type of dressing method on the wound.

Patient（Man）：What do you suggest we use?

Nurse (Woman): Er. I'd like to use a VAC dressing on this wound.

Patient (Man): Oh, sounds nasty.

Nurse (Woman): Mr. Jones. it's called a VAC, which means Vacuum Assisted Closure, but its only a gentle suction on the wound.

Patient (Man): I see. Do you think its a good idea to try that instead of the dressing that they are using now?

Nurse (Woman): Yes. I think it'll help the wound heal faster.

Patient (Man): All right. Sounds like a good idea.

Nurse (Woman): Would you mind if I covered your wound with a dressing towel for now, while I set up the new dressing?

Patient (Man): No, no, I don't mind. Take your time.

Pause (5 seconds)

Repeat

Pause (5 seconds)

This is the end of Part Two.

Pause (5 seconds)

Now look at Part Three.

You will hear a conversation between Helen, the ward nurse, and Mr. Albiston, about his medication.

For questions 11−15, choose the correct answer A, B or C. Put a tick (√) in the box. Then mark the corresponding letter on your answer sheet.

You will hear the conversation twice.

Pause (5 seconds)

Nurse (Woman): Hello, Mr. Albiston. How are you feeling?

Patient (Man): Not too bad, Helen. They started me on a new tablet, I think.

Nurse (Woman): That's right. The doctor's started you on atorvastatin, so I thought I'd have a chat with you, as there are a few things you need to know about it.

Patient (Man): OK. What do I have to know?

Nurse (Woman): The medication is used to prevent atherosclerosis, or clogging of the arteries with fatty deposits.

Patient (Man): I understand.

Nurse (Woman): You take the medication once a day.

Patient (Man): Oh, right. Does it take long to work?

Nurse (Woman): No. it works quite quickly. I've brought a diagram to help you understand what happens when you take this medication. After you swallow the tablet it enters the gastrointestinal tract, or GIT. It passes through the esophagus into your stomach here, where it's absorbed. It then goes into the liver viathe small intestine.

Patient (Man): That's this part under the stomach, isn't it? And it goes across to the liver over here?

Nurse (Woman): Yes. The drug is metabolized, or chemically changed, in the liver. The liver stops the production of an enzyme which causes the body to produce a harmful

135

type of cholesterol. By inhibiting this enzyme, the amount of "bad cholesterol" which is released into the blood is reduced.

Atorvastatin also increases the amount of good cholesterol in your body. This is a protective form of cholesterol.

Patient (Man): I see. So that's why the doctor asked me if I had any problems with my liver. Is it better to take it at night or in the morning?

Nurse (Woman): Take it in the morning. because its absorbed better in the morning than in the evening.

Patient (Man): OK, I'll remember that.

Pause (5 *seconds*)

Repeat

Pause (5 *seconds*)

This is the end of Part Three.

Pause (5 *seconds*)

Now look at Part Four.

You will hear a nurse getting personal details from a patient.

Listen and complete questions 16 – 20 *on your answer sheet.*

You will hear the conversation twice.

Nurse (Woman): Well, have you got an ID bracelet on. Mr. Connolly?

Patient (Man): Yes, here it is.

Nurse (Woman): I just need to check your personal details. Can I look at your ID bracelet, please?

Patient (Man): Yes.

Nurse (Woman): Can you tell me your full name. please?

Patient (Man): It's Stephen Connolly.

Nurse (Woman): Yes, that's S-T-E-P-H-E-N. That's correct on the bracelet. What's your date of birth, please?

Patient (Man): The 30th of November, 1934.

Nurse (Woman): 30th of November,1934. right. Now your hospital number is 463817. I'll just check that on the identity bracelet, 463817. Oh. right. One more question. Do you have any allergies?

Patient (Man): Yes, I do. I'm allergic to morphine. It makes me very sick.

Nurse (Woman): Oh. If you are allergic to something, you should have a red d identity bracelet. I'll change that for you right away.

Patient (Man): Oh, thanks. I forgot to tell them about the allergies.

Nurse (Woman): That's OK, Mr. Connolly. That's why we'd like to check everything carefully. I'll just recheck your pulse first of all. That's fine. It's quite normal, 64 per minute.

Patient(Man): Er, right.

Nurse (Woman): Now your blood pressure. Fine. That's quite normal, too. 130 over 80.

Patient(Man): Oh, I'm pleased to hear it.

Pause（5 seconds）

Repeat

Pause（5 seconds）

This is the end of Part Four.

You now have five minutes to write your answers on the answer sheet.

Pause（4 minutes）

You have one more minute.

Pause（60 seconds）

This is the end of the listening test.

参考文献

［1］段功香.基础护理学实践教程.北京：清华大学出版社,2011.

［2］胡雁.儿科护理学.北京：人民卫生出版社,2005.

［3］姜安丽.护理学基础.北京：人民卫生出版社,2005.

［4］朗文出版公司.朗文当代英语辞典(英语版).北京：外语教学与研究出版社,1997.

［5］李正亚.医护英语水平考试(二级)应考大全.上海：上海外语教育出版社,2016.

［6］林速容.医学英语(Medical English).上海：复旦大学出版社,2016.

［7］刘国全.护理专业英语——视听说分册.北京：人民卫生出版社,2006.

［8］刘国全.护理专业英语——视听说分册学习指导.北京：人民卫生出版社,2006.

［9］王文秀,王颖.护理英语会话.北京：人民卫生出版社,2015.

［10］殷磊.护理学基础.北京：人民卫生出版社,2002.

［11］张银萍,徐红.妇产科护理学.北京：人民卫生出版社,2006.